One-Eyed Princess

Gaining depth in sight and mind

Susanna Zaraysky

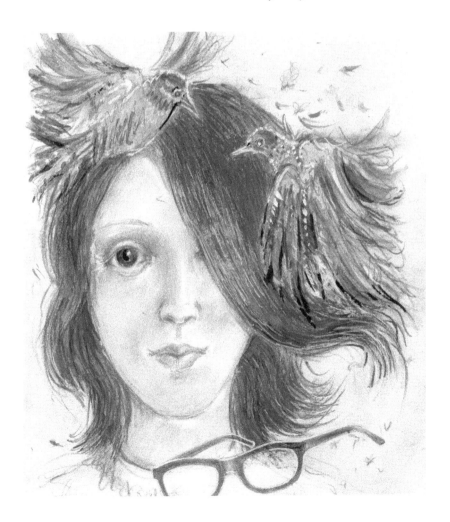

Kaleidomundi
PO Box 1253
Cupertino, CA 95015
USA

www.createyourworldbooks.com
Email: info@kaleidomundi.com

ISBN: 978-0-9820189-1-0
LCCN: 2015913139

Graphic Design by Ivaylo Todorov
Cover Illustration by Valerij Zhelyazkov
Edited by Rachel Banderob and Jonnie Pekelny
Typefaces used in this book are credited as follows:
Hoefler Text and Requem by Hoefler & Co., Myriad Pro by Adobe Systems Inc.

Permissions

Images:

Music lyrics:

Dedications

Since reading about Professor Sue Barry's acquisition of 3D vision in the article "Stereo Sue" by Dr. Oliver Sacks in June 2006 in *The New Yorker* magazine, my life has not been the same. This book is dedicated to both Professor Barry and Dr. Sacks.

Professor Sue Barry, Professor of Neuroscience at Mt. Holyoke College

I have recommended Barry's book, *Fixing My Gaze*, to many people, including to my former ophthalmologist. Sue Barry had the courage to speak up about her changing vision, even though it went against what she had learned in her studies of neuroscience.

Dr. Barry has been a major personal and scientific support for me even before I embarked on this journey to change my brain. We have communicated by postal mail, phone and in person. She even came to my presentation at Google in Mountain View, California about endangered language preservation! Without her, I don't know how I would have undertaken this endeavor. I have communicated with many other amblyopes whose lives have been forever changed since Sue Barry shared her journey. Hopefully, my story can do the same.

Dr. Oliver Sacks, Doctor of Neurology

It was my goal for Dr. Sacks to see this dedication to him before his death in August 2015. (I did write to him and his assistant in February 2015 to let them know I was writing this book and that it would be dedicated to Dr. Sacks.)

When I found out about his death, I fell into a sorrow I had never felt for someone I had never met. If it weren't for Dr. Sacks' work, I would not be the person I am today. I can't think of anyone else whom I have never met who has had such a deep impact on my life. As I learned about the power of music on the brain in Dr. Sacks' book, *Musicophilia*, and realized that I learned languages like songs, I wrote the book, *Language is Music* to help others learn foreign languages in a fun way with music and the media. *Language is Music*, was also dedicated to Dr. Sacks.

Doctors have a direct impact on our lives by listening to our descriptions of our ailments and by treating us with herbs, medicines, therapies, medical devices or by operating on us with surgical implements. It is rare, I believe, to be a patient via words alone. I felt like I was his patient through his articles, books, television interviews, and the movies *Awakenings* and *The Music Never Stopped*, borne out of his writings.

After reading *The New Yorker* article "Stereo Sue," I sent Dr. Oliver Sacks a letter via postal mail. (At the time, he didn't receive emails.) When I received a personal response typed by him, with corrections made by hand, I was deeply moved that he'd taken the time to write back to me and even call me by the moniker I had made for myself, the "One-Eyed Princess." He forwarded my email address to Professor Sue Barry, who wrote to me by email and gave suggestions about vision therapy.

May the legacy of Dr. Sacks touch the lives of many more around the world!

Thanks to you both for your support and for revealing how incredibly the brain can change!

Acknowledgements

There are many people who were key in supporting me in my vision therapy journey and in writing this book.

Jessica Arguëllo did not let me cave into my doubts about publishing this book and revealing the difficulties I experienced as I worked to change my brain. She pressed me to go beyond my fears.

My family was of major support for my journey.

Alexander and Natalie Lara are my nephew and niece, my assistants (a.k.a. "butt kickers") and my vision therapy play buddies. Thank you for providing the fun, laughter and kicks in the butt to do my vision therapy homework.

My parents, Isak and Rimma Zaraysky, and sister Asya Zaraysky, for listening to my trials and tribulations in this process.

My strabismic aunts, Sveta Kanevsky and Lilia Zaraysky, both understood the difficulties I was experiencing and shared their own stories with me. Sveta read several drafts of this book and suggested changes.

Fellow amblyope, César Vasconcelos lent a sympathetic ear and told me of his vision therapy stories. He inspired me with his post-vision therapy tennis prowess.

Dr. Pia Hoenig of the University of California at Berkeley (UC Berkeley) University Eye Center for carefully listening to my issues as I spoke through my tears and giving advice on how to proceed with vision therapy.

Suzanne Bregman for reading the first, second and third drafts of this book and giving me detailed comments and suggestions on how to improve it and for providing me support and comedic distractions in the lab.

My friend, Sarah, was the first and only person to encourage me to do vision therapy. She has been a constant source of support and encouragement.

Elisa Gollub and Scott Neft housed me in their home on many occasions as I went to appointments at UC Berkeley. Elisa also reviewed a draft of this book, giving me helpful feedback on needed changes.

Seema Bhangar and Jim Downing let me stay with them and be entertained by their son, Rohan, on my many trips to Berkeley.

Emanuele Ziglioli, Maren Amdal and Vivian Chong commented on the first rough draft of the book.

Elizabeth Mulford provided me with a sanctuary of solitary splendor where I could write and edit. She also edited the last draft of the book with zeal!

Paulina Novo hosted me on her couch on that fateful trip to Washington DC, where I first learned about seeing in 3D.

Dilip Menon chaperoned me to my vision therapy evaluation on my birthday!

The UC Berkeley Levi lab, where I have been doing computer-based exercises since March 2014, has been a rich environment for me to work on my depth perception and meet fellow amblyopes. Thank you to Dr. Roger Li for accepting me into his study, *An Active Approach to Treat Amblyopia: Perceptual Learning and Video Games* (https://clinicaltrials.gov/ct2/show/NCT01115283) and for carefully taking the time to explain what was going on with my eyes and brain. Michelle Antonucci, John Bui, Ka Yee So and Kenneth D. Tran have patiently listened to me explain my vision. Kenneth worked with me on the definitions section of this book. Ben, although you stole the video game controller from me, your excitement and comments made me smile!

The commenters to my blog helped me feel that I was not alone in my path and struggles to see in 3D. Thanks to Anastasia Burke-Miller (Commenter #14) for sharing her own stories of losing her vision and regaining it to show how flexible our brains are.

Contents

Timeline

Born: with crossed eyes (both eyes were crossed)

Age 3: surgery to straighten eyes, leaves me with a "lazy" eye

Age 15: start to wear contact lenses, eye turn is now obvious (the glasses hid the eye turn before)

Age 17: second surgery leaves eyes cosmetically looking straight, but still vertically and horizontally asymmetric

Age 28: read "Stereo Sue" in *The New Yorker* about Sue Barry, born strabismic and developed 3D vision in her late 40s. The first time I find out I can't see in 3D.

Age 33: start binocular **vision therapy**. See glimpses of 3D using peripheral vision

Notes:

The words in bold are defined in the glossary at the end of the book.

This book is not in chronological order. The sections and chapters are thematic to show how aspects of my vision and life developed.

The names of some people have been changed for privacy reasons.

Introduction

Long before I had ever heard of vision therapy or realized I had a form of blindness called stereo-blindness, Massimo, an Italian chef sitting next to me at an Italian wine and food tasting dinner, told me about the book *A Fortune Teller Told Me* by the Italian author Tiziano Terzani.

"*Devi leggere questo libro* (You have to read this book)," Massimo said.

"*Ma perché?* (But why?)," I asked.

"*Perché sei appassionata della vita* (Because you're impassioned by life)," Massimo responded.

The book was so engrossing that I turned off both my home and mobile phones for an entire weekend to devour it in silence. Over the coming years, Massimo fed me more of Terzani's books. The last book, *La fine è il mio inizio* (*The end is my beginning*), about Terzani's journey with cancer, would illuminate my future awakening in developing depth perception.

Using his language skills (Chinese, Italian, French, German and English), Terzani was always writing dispatches on the lives of other people and explaining the East to the West. After working as a veteran Asian correspondent for the German magazine *Die Spiegel* for decades, Terzani left his globetrotting life and career to take care of himself and grow spiritually in his final years before dying of cancer. He saw his cancer not as a plague, but as a way to travel inside himself. He consulted with many healers, from cancer specialists in the US to spiritual healers in the Philippines, to see if they could cure him. In the end, his cancer gave him a way to understand himself and the meaning of his life.

Although my **amblyopia** and **strabismus** are not fatal diseases, the journey you will read about forced me not only to stop suppressing my vision and strive to see a third dimension of life, but also to develop insight into the dimensions inside of me that I was suppressing.

By improving my **visual acuity** and depth perception, I saw my life anew. Scared, excited, confused and upset, I traveled through a rainbow of emotions by forcing my eyes to work together.

Purposes of this book:

1. To raise awareness of what it is like to live with limited depth perception and rewire one's brain via binocular vision therapy.

2. Hopefully, my showing the personal and emotional journey I traveled to see in depth and gain better visual acuity will help those who face this challenge and those whom they love.

For this book to be understandable to both those with limited depth perception and those with 3D vision, it's important to describe the 2D experience. Like a woman working in a man's world who has had to learn how men think and operate or a left-handed person who has adapted, by force, to a right-handed world by using products meant for right-handed people, those of us with limited depth perception have had to acclimate to a 3D world. However, most people who see in 3D can't understand the limitations of our vision.

While not everyone reading this book will share in the intensity of my experience, I want to help prepare other people who have amblyopia and strabismus for some of the challenges they may have to face should they decide to undertake vision therapy to increase their depth perception. It is important to know that not every stereoblind person has the capacity for stereovision. Eye doctors are still not able to predict how much stereovision a person can acquire via vision therapy. There are amblyopes who have not done vision therapy who see in more depth than I do, even though I have been doing vision therapy for over five years. Patients have different starting points, goals and outcomes.

Additionally, I seek to educate those who have always seen in 3D and can't fathom what life is like for their family, friends and coworkers who have little or no binocular vision so that they can be more sensitive to our limitations.

A few years into the therapy, I realized that I had been going through a grieving process. Unaware that the feelings of frustration and sadness I was experiencing were typical for a person grieving, I struggled with how these emotions impacted my life. I share about this process to aid those who may encounter strong emotions as they work to improve their vision. For those of us who are doing this therapy as adults, we may be peeling away at past trauma and other pain. This road has its benefits but it can be surprisingly difficult along the way.

Before doing vision therapy, I was told that I might experience double vision. However, no medical professional alerted me to other side effects and personal grieving process that dramatically turned my life upside down psychologically, physically, socially and professionally.

I wish I had been told of these side effects:

1. Extreme fatigue.
2. Terrible headaches that could last from one day to the next.
3. Mental confusion, lack of focus.
4. Language confusion.
5. Serious noise sensitivity.
6. Need for social isolation.
7. Difficulty making sense of the world as a result of double vision.
8. Difficulty driving, especially at night.

9. Difficulty driving with double vision.

Most of all, I wished I knew how to communicate what was happening to others.

If you experience some or all of the side effects and changes to your vision and other senses, you are not alone and you are not crazy.

This book is not prescriptive.

Some adults in vision therapy do not experience as many debilitating side effects as I did and some have better results than I did. If I had known what could possibly happen to me, I would have avoided years of frustration and pain. There was no way to avoid the side effects, but I could have prevented some of the psychological and social struggles I went through as I tried desperately to educate those around me about how I was seeing and what I was feeling. I hope this book will help others avert the suffering I experienced.

Rewiring my brain to see in depth impacted almost every area of my life, including the one for which I am best known: being multilingual. I am passionate about language learning and I speak eight languages: English, Russian, French, Spanish, Italian, Portuguese, Bosnian (Serbo-Croatian) and Ladino. I wrote a book on foreign language learning using music and the media, called *Language is Music*, which has been translated into Portuguese, Russian and Spanish. To my stunned surprise, (as I explain in Chapter Three), as a result of changing my brain, even speaking in English became difficult.

Proverb:
In the land of the blind, the one-eyed man is king.

In the land of the stereoblind, the one-eyed person is normal.

In the land of not knowing oneself, the one-eyed person who has gone through binocular vision therapy and has reached deep inside to acquire self-knowledge, reigns.

I am the one-eyed princess.

Definitions, wording

In this book, I refer to myself and others with amblyopia and other vision conditions who see in 2D as living in "flatland" or in a "2D world." It's not that our lives are so flat that we live on paper like the kind this book is printed on or that our lives are boring and deficient because we don't see in 3D. I use these terms as markers of what it is to see the world with limited depth. We all inhabit the same world, whether we see it in 3D or 2D. I also use the word "normal" to refer to people who are binocular, have straight eyes and see in 3D because this is the term people often used to compare my situation to what people know to be standard. I don't use this term to be self-deprecating, it's simply an easy reference point for people to understand.

There is a spectrum of binocularity. Not everyone with amblyopia and/or strabismus sees with the same amount of limited depth perception that I do: some see more and some see less.

If you're an amblyope, you may resonate with some of my descriptions and not with others because you may see more or less depth than I do. These descriptions are verbal illustrations of what I have seen and not definitive definitions of how one should see.

Since I do not see in 3D, I cannot provide a super clear comparison of 3D vs 2D vision. I can only use the words and explanations I've learned over the years to describe my reality. For a comparison of 3D and 2D vision from people who have seen the world with both types of vision, please read the descriptions of the books *Fixing My Gaze* and *The Mind's Eye* at the end of this book.

What are amblyopia, strabismus, and vision therapy? There is a glossary at the end of this book with more definitions.

Amblyopia (pronounced: amblee-o-pee-ah) (also called lazy eye) is a disorder of sight. This is a developmental problem that results as a compensating mechanism to prevent diplopia. As a result, there is decreased vision in one eye that is usually independent of anatomical damage in the eye or visual pathways. This is correctable if caught early. This is usually uncorrectable by eyeglasses or contact lenses.

There are five types of amblyopia: deprivation amblyopia (from congenital cataracts present at birth), anisometropic, meridional, refractive and strabismic amblyopia.

It involves decreased vision in an eye that otherwise appears normal.

In amblyopia, visual stimulation either fails to be or is poorly transmitted through the optic nerve to the brain for a continuous period of time. It can also occur when the brain "turns off" the visual processing of one eye to prevent double-vision, for example in strabismus (crossed eyes). It often occurs during early childhood and results in poor or blurry vision.

Some people have a very small asymmetry in their eyes, so you may not be able to detect it. Some of us have had operations to cosmetically straighten our eyes so we appear "normal." The small asymmetry that we do have in our eyes is imperceptible to most people.

Before I learned the medical definition of amblyopia, I always thought that amblyopia was for someone with a "lazy eye"; however, I only recently learned that I was wrong. Not all amblyopes have squints or asymmetric eyes. Some amblyopes have vastly different acuity in each eye and the brain can't fuse the images from the two eyes. One eye could be myopic and the other **far-sighted**; therefore images don't double but the image in the far-sighted eye is bigger than what the **near-sighted** eye perceives. I wonder what it is like for someone with one far-sighted eye and another near sighted eye to look at an object, first with one eye and then with the other, and see it a different size. In addition to the segment of the population with amblyopia, there are people who have limited or no vision in one of their eyes and they also have no or very little depth perception. There are people with binocular vision issues due to strokes, brain trauma or loss of sight in one eye.

Strabismus (pronounced: strah-biz-mus), or crossed eyes, is the inability to direct both eyes towards the same fixation point. One eye may appear to turn in (esotropia), out (exotropia), up (hypertropia), or down (hypotropia). The eye turn may occur constantly or only intermittently. Eye-turning may change from one eye to the other (alternating strabismus), and may appear only when a person is tired or has done a lot of reading (decompensated phoria). Strabismus may cause double vision. To avoid seeing dou-

ble, vision in one eye may be ignored or suppressed resulting in a lazy eye (amblyopia).

Strabismus is a condition in which the eyes are not properly aligned with each other. It typically involves a lack of coordination between the extraocular muscles, which prevents bringing the gaze of each eye to the same point in space, which thus hampers proper binocular vision, and which may adversely affect depth perception.

Amblyopia is a condition caused by strabismus (or other amblyogenic factors).

Vision therapy (VT) *is a type of physical therapy for the eyes and brain. It is a non-surgical treatment for many common visual problems such as lazy eye, crossed eyes, double vision,* **convergence insufficiency** *and some reading and learning disabilities.*

I use the acronym VT throughout the book to refer to vision therapy for amblyopia and strabismus. When I refer to VT patients, I am writing about patients undergoing vision therapy for amblyopia and strabismus and not other conditions.

Why I wrote this book even though at first I didn't want to do it

I wish I didn't have to write this book. I wish this book, or a version of it, had already been written before I had embarked on vision therapy.

What prompted me to compose this book was the scarcity of information available about what it is like to live without 3D vision and what it is like to change one's brain in the pursuit of improved depth perception. According to the American Optometric Association, it is estimated that two to four percent of the population has amblyopia[1]. The American Association for Pediatric Ophthalmology and Strabismus states that about four percent of the population has a form of strabismus[2]. If we take an average and say 3% of the population has one or both of the conditions, then that means that one out of 33 people can't see in 3D. Despite the fact that we are not unique "one in a million" cases, few people know that our hidden disability exists. When I told people, even medical professionals who were not eye doctors, that I could not see in 3D, they looked at me dumbfounded. They had never met anyone else who had told them that they saw the world in 2D. Even if they closed one eye, they might not have approximated 2D vision because their brain would fill in the missing information from the closed eye.

I was showered with questions:

How can you survive?

How can you step down from the curb on the street if you can't see the distance between the curb and the street?

How can you drive?

Do I look flat to you, like people on TV?

The question about "looking flat" like on TV seemed so silly to me because for years, as a kid, my parents had a black and white TV. When we got a color TV, it didn't have cable, so many images were not sharp. So of course people in real life weren't in black and white and/or fuzzy! I truly had never thought about the difference between "real life" images and TV. They actually

---

1 "It is estimated that two to four percent of children have amblyopia." http://www.aoa.org/patients-and-public/eye-and-vision-problems/glossary-of-eye-and-vision-conditions/amblyopia/amblyopia-faqs?sso=y
2 " It is estimated that 4% of the U.S. population has strabismus." http://www.aapos.org/terms/conditions/100

didn't seem that different, as long as the TV image was of high quality. Of course I knew that people and objects on TV weren't as flat as the television screen and that the news announcer was not part of the wall behind him or her but that was obvious. Why were people asking me such a dumb question?

The more I tried to explain my vision, the more I understood why people asked me such silly, and sometimes offensive, questions. They had no idea what I was talking about.

How could my situation be so novel to others if I was one of millions worldwide? Obviously, everyone I told knew more than just 33 people. There was no way I was the only person they knew with amblyopia or strabismus.

The issue was not that I was alone. I was just one of few individuals who openly spoke about not seeing with both eyes. When I first started VT in January 2010, I didn't know of other VT bloggers. My only point of reference was Dr. Sue Barry. Then, I saw a few more bloggers writing about their experiences and I found a couple Yahoo groups on VT and strabismus and an online community of both practitioners and people undergoing VT. But still, there were few resources for support.

I met other adult strabismics in person and online who had NEVER met anyone else like them with the same problem. How is this possible if approximately one in every 33 people has amblyopia and/or strabismus?

Some people live in shame because of jokes about their divergent eyes as kids. If they're like me and can pass as "normal" (due to surgery, minor asymmetry or because their eyes are straight but have vastly different acuity), they may be thrilled to not be made fun of anymore and they may not want to bring up the subject. The brother of a close friend of mine who lives in Mumbai, India wrote to me asking me about my therapy. He is also strabismic. Mumbai has about 13 million people; if 3% of them have amblyopia that means around 390,000 people in his city have it. Nonetheless, he had to write to me, halfway across the world, to communicate from the heart about his vision problems. When he and I met in Berkeley, California, I took him to the lab where I undergo vision therapy. He quickly felt eye strain when doing the computer exercises and playing 3D video games. He was surprised to find out from me that head tilting was a common trait. He'd been wondering his whole life why he tilted his head and strained his neck. The head tilting, as I came to learn when I found out that I often tilted my head, is common for those with asymmetric eyes because we move our heads to a position where we avoid double vision and can see straight. It was a relief for him to speak to me about his eyes.

I calculated that in the 25 or so houses on my street, there were probably 100 residents. There might be two other amblyopes on my street. Yet I felt incredibly alone.

Thirty or forty years ago, teachers and parents might have thought dyslexic kids were slow or stupid. Now we know that kids with dyslexia need special assistance reading because their brains switch letters around, resulting in reading problems. This doesn't mean that every dyslexic student gets special help and none fall through the cracks of our educational system, but at least the word "dyslexia" is a household term. Most people have some idea of what the disability is and understand that a dyslexic kid has trouble reading.

What I want is for amblyopia and strabismus (or at least the terms "lazy eye" and "crossed eyes") to also be household terms so that parents, teachers and medical professionals are sensitive to the needs of people who can't see in depth.

It is crucial to have early identification of binocularity issues by **optometrists** in schools. If children and parents know early-on that there is a problem seeing with both eyes, then the parent can look into which options are best for the child. Some parents falsely assume that if their child can read or pass a simple eye exam by reading an eye chart, that the child has normal vision. I had read eye charts for years at the doctor's office and at the Department of Motor Vehicles when getting a driver's license. Nonetheless, I had no idea that I couldn't see with both eyes.

I hope that this book, in addition to helping amblyopic adults know what it could be like to change their brains to see in depth, will help amblyopic children and parents navigate what may be ahead of them with doctors, treatments, emotional trauma and personal development. Being looked at funny and taunted by kids because of one's asymmetric eyes can have lifelong repercussions, leading the amblyope to constantly feel self-conscious about their looks and shy away from social interaction. Some amblyopic children struggle with reading and other activities and may be put in remedial reading classes in school for the wrong reasons. Parents of amblyopic children may be pulling their hair out trying to comprehend the struggles their children are going through. These parents may not understand why their kids can't play tennis and are terrified of driving. They may push their children to do things they are not meant or able to do or with which they need extra help.

By educating about the impact of living with 2D vision, this book may reduce the ignorance around the condition and sensitize people.

There is no intent to embarrass or shame those whose actions and insensitivity have caused me frustration or pain. Those actions were not borne out of malice, but out of ignorance and carelessness. I have exposed my emotional journey to help those with normal vision to understand the emotional and practical consequences of their failure to understand, remember or take into account the limitations faced by the stereo blind. My accounts may also serve as a warning to those with limited depth perception to reduce their level of frustration when their friends and family do not understand their struggles.

What finally compelled me to publish my anonymous blog into a book with my name

I had my blog under the URL www.oneeyedprincess.com for several years without my name on it. I wanted my writings to be anonymous while at the same time connecting with others who had the condition or who were family members of those with amblyopia and strabismus. I didn't want my name to be known.

My blog was one of my few outlets for expressing how my life really was.

On my fourth year anniversary of being in VT, two famous men, a mustached dead painter and a living music star, inspired me to break my silence.

As a birthday present to myself, I bought a ticket for the concert of my favorite musician, Billy Joel. I flew from California to Tampa, Florida, just to attend his concert. Joel had been my favorite singer since I was in elementary school and it was my first time seeing him live. Before Joel had agreed to the concert tour, he firmly said he wasn't just going to play his "hits," he was going to perform whatever songs he wanted.

At age 64, Billy Joel filled the stadium. Some people were standing. Who else in their 60s besides him, Mick Jagger, Paul McCartney, Roger Waters and maybe Barbara Streisand could fill a stadium of 22,000 people? His star power was stronger than that of many world leaders. At his age and at this point in his career, he could play whatever he wanted and his concerts would still sell out. When Billy Joel composed his songs, he didn't write them with the intention of all of his songs becoming hits. He wrote the pieces from the heart, making his lyrics so sincere and painful. I didn't want to wait until I was 64 to have the courage to speak my mind, even if people around me didn't understand.

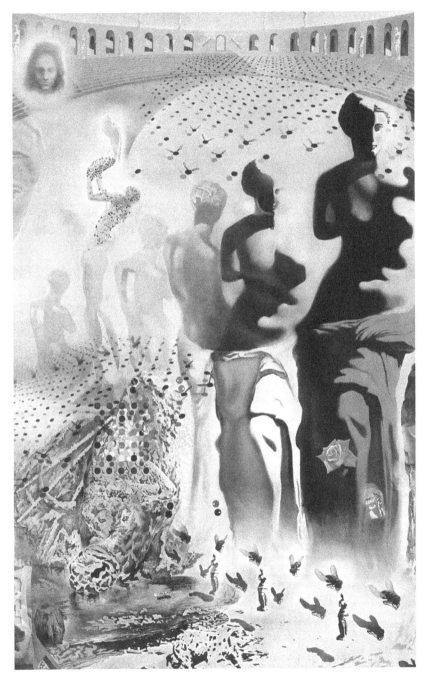

Salvador Dalí, "Hallucinogenic Toreador"
Image credit: © Salvador Dalí, Fundació Gala-Salvador Dalí, Artists Rights
Society (ARS), New York 2015

Two days after the concert, and exactly four years after I had started vision therapy, I saw my double vision problems visually represented, on the canvas of a major painter! I went to the Dalí Museum in the Florida city eponymous with the city of my birth, St. Petersburg.

While I had never been a fan of Salvador Dalí's work, two friends had recommended I visit the museum since I was going to be in the area. The bullfighter on the Venus de Milo statues in the painting pictured in the "Hallucinogenic Toreador" painting struck me. I might not have noticed the double image if it had not been for the explanation of the audio guide. (Clues: There are two bullfighters transposed on top of the right two Venus de Milo statues. The bullfighter's tie is on the bottom part of the second Venus de Milo's robe.)

I was so happy to see something representing my distorted vision. Awestruck, I listened to the audio guide explain the images of the bull fighters on the bodies of the Venus de Milo statues. This is what it is like sometimes when I see in double: I see one image juxtaposed onto another image and I have to remind myself which object or person is real and which is a phantom image created in my brain.

When Dalí presented his work, people might have thought he was crazy. According to Dalí, his professors at La Real Academia de Bellas Artes de San Fernando (*Royal Academy of Fine Arts of San Fernando*) in Madrid, Spain, didn't appreciate his work. But his professors aren't in every art book. Dalí is.

I realized that no matter how alienating it was to communicate about my improved vision and distortions, I had to do it, even if most people wouldn't understand me in the slightest.

Finally I can tell people who don't understand 2D vision and double vision, "I sometimes see like the double images in Dalí's paintings"! Having the Dalí reference is monumental. Previously, when I had seen his work in books, I just thought he was a weird painter whom I couldn't understand. Now I appreciate that he showed the world how some of us with intermittent diplopia see and struggle to explain it to others.

I was ecstatic at the museum but I had no one with whom to comment. I didn't feel comfortable telling the other museum visitors, "I sometimes see the world like a Dalí invention!"

When I returned home, I told my friends about how inspired I was by Joel and Dalí to communicate no matter what others may say or not understand.

While connecting to other adults with my same condition and those doing VT, I found that we had similar difficulties and perceptions of life. This helped me feel less isolated. I discovered that my noise sensitivity seemed to be common amongst other adults doing VT. Several people who had successfully crossed from 2D to 3D said that once they could see in 3D, they felt more like they were a part of their surroundings. Previously, with 2D vision, they felt that they had been merely observing their surroundings while seeing in 2D. Since I have yet to cross the threshold into 3D, I can't echo these sentiments, but I do know that I have felt like an observer all my life. This could be due to many factors, including being from an immigrant family and living in many countries, where I had to observe others to understand how to act and speak. It could be that those of us who were made fun of as children because of our odd looking eyes felt less comfortable being the center of attention and preferred to be on the sidelines or do things on our own to avoid people making comments about our eyes or looking at us funny. This may also explain why there are several artists who are amblyopes who have written to Dr. Sue Barry. Artists have to be keen observers of life in order to transpose what they see onto a canvas, a 2D art form.

One VT blogger took a poll asking how many of us adult amblyopes had low blood pressure. It turns out that in her pool of respondents, low blood pressure was a common theme. Both of my strabismic aunts have low blood pressure, as do I. When I told this to my first developental optometrist, he said that there was no correlation between our eye condition and blood pressure. Nonetheless, it makes me wonder what other medical conditions we may share. If more of us talk about these common traits, we could help researchers understand more about the condition and how it affects other aspects of our bodies.

I thought that by expanding on my blog and revealing my story in this book, I could help amblyopes understand that their anti-social behavior, feelings of being an outsider, or other medical conditions are shared amongst others just like them.

I want other amblyopes to feel comfortable telling people why they can't park, drive, play tennis, or walk down stairs quickly and have their friends say, "Oh yes, I know of amblyopia. I understand that you can't see in depth. Tell me, what can I do to be of service to you?" Perhaps this book may inspire people to make assistive technologies for those with limited depth perception.

My story is a personal account of what it was like for me as a child, teenager and adult before I pursued vision therapy to develop 3D vision and how my life has changed since I chose to undertake binocular vision therapy.

DISCLAIMER

I am writing from my own experience to share my journey about how my hidden disability and my journey to improve my vision gave me a new perspective on life. This book does not claim to represent everyone with 2D vision or every vision therapy patient. I do not represent any optometry, vision therapy or ophthalmology associations, nor was this book commissioned by anyone or any organization.

Frequently Asked Questions

Q: Have I expended many financial resources on vision therapy?

A: Yes.

Q: Have I awakened crying every day for several months wondering when I'll finally see in 3D and hoping my side effects will go away?

A: Yes.

Q: Have I felt deep frustration after realizing that no matter how much I explain to family and friends about my vision, they still don't get it and continue to say and do insensitive things?

A: Yes.

Q: Do I regret dedicating over five years of my life to improving my vision and changing my brain?

A: Absolutely not.

What I have learned about myself and how we perceive "reality" is something I would have never picked up in books, a self-development class or from a guru. I learned it because vision therapy has not only improved how I see the world around me but it made me see myself and how I relate to people in a completely new and enriched way. For these new insights, I am very grateful to Dr. Oliver Sacks who first "opened" my eyes to vision therapy when I read about Sue Barry in his *New Yorker* article, "Stereo Sue." (See more about this book in the Resources section at the end.)

What is a hidden (or invisible) disability?

It is important to understand that people with amblyopia and strabismus may share similar struggles with other people who also have hidden handicaps. Not all hidden disabilities affect people in the same way or have the same level of severity; some can be intensely disruptive on a chronic basis while others can be mild or acute.

Amblyopia and strabismus, especially for those whose eyes appear to be straight or are straight, are hidden disabilities because the outside world does not perceive us as disabled. However, what we all share is that we have a condition others can't see and therefore may not appreciate.

...

When you see someone on crutches, do you feel a need to offer assistance?

When they near a door, do you motion to open the door for them?

When they enter a room, do you consider giving up your seat or bringing them what they need?

If an elderly or disabled person boards a bus, typically someone at the front of the bus gives them their seats.

Would you do the same?

I hope the answers to all of those questions are yes.

There is compassion in the world for elderly or disabled persons.

Do you know of someone with a hidden disability?

Someone who describes their challenges, but has no outward appearance of being disabled? Is it fairly easy to forget their disability because you cannot see it? And since you can't see it, how easy is it to question its existence? Is it awkward to consider how best to accommodate them?

Living with a hidden disability is like living with crutches—but you just can't see them.

While there are more, here are some hidden disabilities you may know:

Anxiety disorders	*Circadian rhythm sleep disorders*	*Irritable Bowel Syndrome*
Allergies		*Lactose Intolerance*
Amblyopia	*Celiac Disease*	*Lyme Disease*
Asperger Syndrome	*Crohn's disease*	*Migraines*
Asthma	*Depression*	*Multiple Sclerosis*
Autism	*Diabetes*	*Narcolepsy*
Bipolar disorder	*Epilepsy*	*Personality disorders*
Brain injuries	*Fibromyalgia*	*Repetitive stress injuries*
Charcot-Marie-Tooth disease	*Food allergies*	*Rheumatoid arthritis*
Chronic fatigue syndrome	*Fructose malabsorption*	*Schizophrenia*
Chronic pain	*Hypoglycemia*	*Strabismus*
	Inflammatory bowel disease	*Temporomandibular joint disorder*

Most likely, you either have one of the conditions listed above or you know someone who does.

This book is about a hidden visual disability and it may resonate with those who have other conditions with invisible symptoms.

It often feels like those of us who struggle with amblyopia are in an "us vs. them" situation, with "them" being binocular people who can't understand us. By explaining this topic to help people understand what it's like to have a hidden disability, I aim to expand the "we" and reduce the "them" camps.

If you can't understand how it is for an amblyope who can only see "flat," think about how your friends who have asthma feel when they can't walk for too long without losing their breath and keep getting invited on long hikes in the mountains by friends who know that they're asthmatic. How isolated do your lactose-intolerant relatives feel when they attend a family meal where all of the food has dairy?

It's hard to step into someone else's shoes, especially when the shoes are invisible. However, if you can think of several people you know with hidden disabilities and combine their symptoms, you are getting closer to empathizing with the amblyope(s) in your life who may need your support.

If you're an amblyope and your friends and family don't understand the limitations of your vision because they assume that you must see like they do since you don't walk with a cane, think of someone they know with a hidden disability. Explain how that other person's hidden disability impacts their life and draw comparisons to your boundaries. While it is hard, and sometimes inappropriate, to compare ailments, it might be a way for your friends and family to understand that something they don't see actually does exist.

CHAPTER ONE

From Developmentally Disabled to Finding a New World

Blog comments:

I've left some of the comments people wrote on my blog posts to show the support and understanding I felt from readers—people who were reading and commenting on my blog because they were going through VT, were VT practitioners, or had children going through the therapy.

Born asymmetric in the former Soviet Union

I was born with wandering eyes, each moving in its own direction, not in coordination with the other.

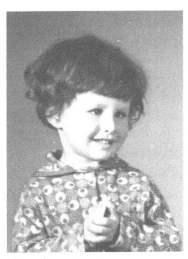

The only day care in Leningrad that would take me was the one for developmentally disabled children. Since I wasn't mentally disabled, I was the only "normal" kid in a daycare of toddlers with developmental disabilities. Maybe this was where I started to understand different forms of

Crossed eyes at age two

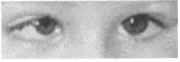

Photos of me circa 2 yrs old

communication, helping me later on to learn various languages. I didn't do any patching on one eye to strengthen the other eye nor did I have any surgeries to straighten my eyes.

Seeing in the dark
St. Louis, Missouri, 1980

My family emigrated to the US from the former USSR in the spring of 1980. The eye doctors at one of the St. Louis hospitals immediately offered a surgery to straighten my crossed eyes, explaining to my parents that the Soviet medical system should have given me stronger glasses when I was younger or performed surgery on my eyes when I was a baby. The surgery I received in St. Louis was not a complete fix as I still had a lazy eye that did not move in sync with the other one. After the surgery, I wore very thick spectacles, jokingly referred to as "Coke bottle glasses" because they were as thick as a glass Coca Cola bottle. They overly magnified my eyes, making them appear to be straight. Therefore, I didn't realize that there was anything wrong with my vision.

Before getting out of bed in the morning and putting on my spectacles, I loved practicing my "supernatural" ability of moving objects with my eyes. Unaware that my eyes weren't coordinated, with one eye seeing an object in one place and the other viewing it in another location, I thought I had a magical power to move the world around. If I looked at an object on my nightstand and then blinked, I moved it to a new place. When I looked at the white ceiling, I saw moving dots of various colors. I was confused because I knew that the ceiling was white, everyone said it was white, but I saw moving colors. I didn't tell anybody about my secret abilities to see colors and move objects.

One of my first memories of living in this new country is that we lived in darkness in the humid hot summer months in Missouri.

My magical vision was less noticeable because I couldn't move objects around if I couldn't see them well in the dark. My family wasn't afraid of the cold winter, but soon after we arrived in the US in May, the Midwestern humidity and heat felt like a death sentence. The weak air conditioner wasn't powerful enough to keep the apartment cool and my parents could not afford a better one. Mom cut up brown paper grocery bags and taped them on the windows and lowered the dark blinds to keep out the heat, making the whole apartment dark. Terribly depressed by the darkness, Mom was reminded of the World War II years in the Soviet Union when her mother had to turn off all of the lights and close the window curtains so that the Nazis would think that the apartment was uninhabited and would not drop a bomb. It was harder for my sister and me to bounce on the bean bags because the humidity made us stick to the vinyl.

My linguistic world was delineated by a chamber of Russian darkness at home and the big-windowed, illuminated and airy English air-conditioned day care. My first time in a school not specifically for the developmentally disabled commenced in English. However, I didn't understand the other kids because they were all speaking in a language I didn't know. I felt alone and confused. Disoriented, I didn't understand the games the kids were playing and the nursery rhymes and songs they were learning. I sat on the light brown wooden, lacquer-covered gymnasium floor and traced my eyes around the painted basketball court's half circles and squares. I looked at the other kids in amazement. I didn't know where I was and what they were saying. I just wanted to be with my family, in our dark, hot apartment with the sticky bean bag chairs. Luckily, there was a Russian-speaking day care teacher who explained to me the drills for tornadoes and the nap-time and snack rules. I didn't understand the Midwestern word "tornado" and got scared when the "tomato" drill bell rang and we had to run for cover. Mom taught me the Russian alphabet at home and helped me with the English alphabet when we were riding the bus to preschool. Eventually I learned English and enjoyed playing with the other kids.

One of the first phrases I understood was "four eyes." Some kids were teasing me for the chunky magnifying glasses resting on the bridge of my nose. I felt ugly and unwanted from their jokes. I didn't tell the kids about my special powers to move objects because I didn't want to bring more attention to my eyesore glasses.

Second surgery

At age 15, I started to wear contact lenses. However, once I put on the lenses, my wander-

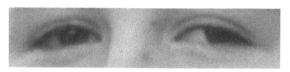

My lazy left eye at age 13

ing eye became very apparent and confused people who were speaking to me. They couldn't tell if I was actually looking at them or somewhere else. Maybe the reason I became such a good listener was so that people would enjoy talking to me and forget about my weird eye. Annoyed at people's confusion and embarrassed to publicly show my painful disability, I fervently wanted to straighten my eyes. My ophthalmologist in Santa Clara, California agreed to perform another operation to straighten my eyes, warning me that this would not be a permanent fix. Eventually, my eyes would diverge again. For six months before the operation, I had to perform eye exercises to strengthen my eye muscles. The vision therapist taught me how to focus one eye on a stick that I held with my hand about a foot (about 30 cm) away from my head and alternate looking at the stick and the wall. Performing this exercise shattered my illusion of being able to move objects. When I told the vision therapist about my "magical power," she laughed and told me that many cross-eyed people have the same thoughts of magical vision. It turns out that I had no special powers! I just couldn't see straight because my eyes saw objects in different places. Objects moved when my brain switched from one eye to another. My magic was actually just my disability.

During my spring vacation when I was 17, I underwent eye surgery that became a major turning point in my life. After the surgery, my eyes looked symmetrical although they still had a vertical and horizontal asymmetry. I could no longer change the positioning of things around me. My magic was gone, but I had more confidence in my appearance. I didn't have to wear my Coke bottle glasses and no one looked at me funny because they couldn't tell if I was paying attention to them. I looked like everyone else. My eye complex was temporarily gone.

There's a third dimension of life that I'm not seeing!
Washington, DC, New York, July 2006

I was visiting my friend Paulina in Washington, DC for the July 4th holiday. Paulina and her roommates let me sleep on the couch in the living room. Her German roommate Sebastian had left an issue of *The New Yorker* on a table near the couch. Unable to fall asleep, I picked up Sebastian's magazine and was intrigued by the title of one of the articles, "Stereo Sue." The author, renowned neurologist Dr. Oliver Sacks, told the story of a cross-eyed woman who had developed stereoptic (three-dimensional) vision in her 40s by doing binocular vision therapy. By doing visual exercises, she learned to coordinate her eyes so her brain would fuse images. I read the article until I was too tired to keep my eyes open. Sebastian allowed me to take the magazine with me back to New York.

While riding the air conditioned New York subway on the way to Grand Central Station to get new contact lenses, my eyes were glued to the magazine. The author stated that describing three-dimensional vision to someone who couldn't see in 3D was like describing color to a blind person. I looked up from the magazine and wondered, "was I as blind to the three-dimensional world as "Stereo Sue" had been?" When "Stereo Sue" developed three-dimensional vision, she spent an hour staring at falling snowflakes. She was in awe of how much more vivid they were than when she had previously seen with just one eye working at a time.

I walked out of Grand Central Station, holding my magazine in one hand and my water bottle in the other. I exited into the humid July heat and looked for my new doctor's office amidst all the scaffolding blocking the names of offices. In a daze of shock from the article, I didn't notice the racks of eyeglass frames in the window and walked right past the optometrist's office. I reached the end of the block and turned back to find the doctor's office.

"Doctor, are you saying that the rest of the world sees a dimension of life that I can't see?" I asked.

Standing a foot away from the examination chair, the optometrist paused.

"Your eyes alternate. Since you don't use them at the same time, your brain doesn't fuse images to create a three-dimensional picture."

"I see flat while the rest of the world sees something I can't even imagine?" I asked.

I was 29 years old and the tears in my eyes were about to burst into a waterfall. I didn't want the doctor to know how shocked and hurt I was. I felt embarrassed that I never knew that despite my two operations, my being born cross-eyed had kept me from seeing the world the same way other people do.

"You don't see completely flat. Your mind picks up on monocular cues to create some sort of depth perception. If it didn't, you'd be dead by now. You would not be able to cross the sidewalk without tripping or drive without crashing your car."

I felt as though my whole life had just turned upside down. Why hadn't my doctors told me earlier that I was unable to see a dimension of life that sounded like it made life look fuller and richer? Why hadn't they told me that vision exercises might help me see that other dimension? More importantly, why hadn't anyone explained to me that my limited blindness could cause me problems in driving and parking—two activities that had been super hard for me?

"My wife's aunt couldn't see the tree outside her window. When I gave her a pair of glasses to improve her far-sightedness, she never wore them. She didn't care to see farther than her window. Maybe you don't need to see in three dimensions. You've gotten this far without it," he said.

I was from California. We had lots of trees in front of our windows in California and I enjoyed looking at them. I wanted to see farther than my window. I had looked through many windows on airplanes, trains, buses, pick-up trucks, vans and cars, and even open-air views from a horse drawn hay cart in rural Romania. I was a globetrotter. My passports had been in 45 countries in the past 20 years—more than many of my compatriots could locate on a map. My bulging passport would need a second set of extra pages to accommodate the stamps for my future international travels. If there was another dimension of the world, I definitely wanted to see it!

I left the office into the humid and polluted Manhattan air, which descended on my salty tear-filled face.

I walked into the delicatessen at the train station and looked at all the gourmet foods and wondered what I was missing. How did everyone else see this $30/pound fancy English cheese? Did these truffles appear more attractive to people who saw with both eyes? I knew what these foods tasted like, but I couldn't fathom how other people saw them. Walking to the subway, I looked at people and they seemed like paper cut-outs. Previously round, curved and shaped, people now manifested into dull figures. They were flat. But they hadn't been flat before I had gone to the eye doctor. The individuals were normal looking, like other people. Now, they were profiles. I realized that I could barely detect the distance between someone's nose and cheeks. It was the shadow from the nose that denoted the space. Oh my! I didn't even know what I looked like to other people! I might look so much different to the rest of the world than I appeared to myself. Maybe the curves around my hips looked less fatty to those who could see with two eyes!

The doctor's words keep ringing in my ears.

"Susanna, you see flat."

"Over ninety five percent of the population can see something you can't see."

I returned home lost in thought. I called my two strabismic aunts and one friend, Jonnie (one of the editors of this book), whom I knew had my same condition. They were all surprised to find out that I had not known I was monocular. I had been in two-dimensional ignorance all these years and had no idea what I was missing.

Was my ignorance my bliss?

At least now I had a valid excuse for being occasionally clumsy. I had answers to issues that had been bothering me for a while. I wasn't just inept at tennis and ping-pong, my eyes were at fault! I couldn't hit the ball because I couldn't judge the ball's distance from me. My lack of depth perception must have accounted for my hatred of merging traffic and parallel parking. I got bored when I read overly detailed descriptions of interiors and locations. Maybe other people put so much thought into characterizing how things looked because they saw something with both eyes that didn't strike me as so compelling when I only saw with one.

After finding out I could only see in 2D, I met a chiropractor in Manhattan's East Village specializing in neurological work who performed coordination tests on me.

"You indeed have poor coordination and concentration due to the fact that your neurological system is only processing information from one eye at a time," he said.

Finally, I had an excuse for messing up in partner dancing! My brain just couldn't keep my eyes and body in rhythm.

Over the coming weeks, I marinated and brewed in my new reality. It was as though I were a piece of furniture absorbing a new varnish. This new coat of color on me was fogging up my world, changing how I perceived reality. Feeling like a captive of my two-dimensional world, I was unable to appreciate the beauty around me. I felt deprived, angry, inferior and distant from other people. How could I explain my reality if what I saw was so drastically different from what most people could perceive? When I told people with 3D vision that I only saw in 2D, their jaws dropped. How could I and a color blind person live in the same world demarcated by distances and color, yet experience it in such vastly different ways? There was no way to prove what a color was or how something looked if some of us were literally blind to various dimensions of life.

What was real?

Though I couldn't prove what was real, I did know that my cursed eyes were actually more of a nuisance than I had ever previously imagined. I had been plagued by my vision issues my entire life. Delighted to be straight eyed and without glasses after my operation at age 17, I had enjoyed several adolescent years of visual bliss. My few golden years had come to a dramatic and painful end on the Danube in 1997. An eye infection I got in Budapest kept me from wearing contacts for several years. I was pained with my thick glasses again until one of my coworkers suggested I get new modern thin lenses. Still, the childhood complex of wearing glasses and having divergent eyes had never left me, no matter how trendy and sleek my frames were. Once my infection went away, I could wear contacts again and have a better image of myself than when I wore glasses. But I still hated being spectacled in any form.

One eye or two? Most painful test I ever took at Berkeley
May 2008

For two years, I thought about vision therapy, but I didn't pursue it for financial reasons. Finally in May 2008, I took the first step to trying VT and made an appointment at the Binocular Vision Clinic at the University of California at Berkeley (UC Berkeley) Optometry Clinic.

I arrived at the Sunnyvale Caltrain station and there were no parking spaces in the train parking lot. Instead, I parked in a municipal lot across the street from the train station and risked getting a parking ticket since the parking lot had a three-hour limit. I parked, ran to the station and arrived breathless to the platform, just in time for my train.

About an hour and a half later, I arrived in Berkeley. While riding the campus shuttle, a fire alarm had sounded and many students were exiting one of the buildings. I joked with the bus driver that probably one of the students was stressed about an exam that day and had pulled the fire alarm to cancel the exam.

Little did I know that I would soon face the most difficult exam I had ever taken on the Berkeley campus. (I had done my undergraduate studies at UC Berkeley.) The test was not just an examination of my eyes and brain, but one of how to maintain my composure. This was my first realization that the journey to binocular vision was one of patience and endurance.

I had been waiting half a year for an appointment in the Binocular Vision Clinic. Getting an appointment was difficult given the small clinic staff. Due to travel, I had had to cancel two previous appointments. Binocular vision specialists are so scarce that some patients even flew in from other states.

I told the resident and intern how the "Stereo Sue" article had turned my world around and how I wanted to know if I could have depth perception. Since I had never used both eyes together, it was possible that my brain had never formed the brain cells to process 3D images and fuse vision.

For an hour and a half, the resident and intern performed many tests on my eyes to see how well they worked together and separately. I had to put on funny plastic **red-green glasses** that had one red and one green lens and look at a red-green eye chart. Half of the letters on the eye chart could be seen through the red lens and the other half, through the green lens. The point of the exercise was to determine if I could see all the letters at the same time through both lenses. Sometimes I could see all of the letters and at other times they would just disappear.

Can things just vanish from one's sight? Yes they can. It's as though they don't even exist.

The real test came when I looked through glass lenses in an **amblyoscope**, a big optometric machine, at a picture of a cat. There were two pictures: the left picture was of a cat with whiskers without a tail and the right one had the cat with a tail, but no whiskers. The aim of the exercise was to see how long my

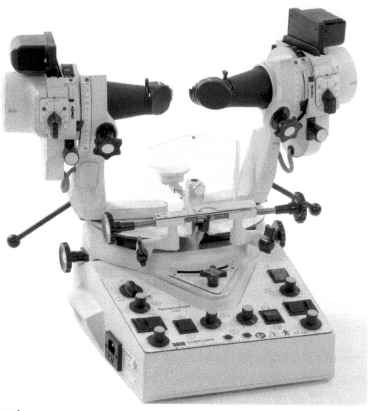

Amblyoscope
Image credit: © *Bernell Corporation*

eyes could work together and let me see a fully bodied feline with both the whiskers and tail. The tail and whiskers came in and out of sight. I remembered the fire alarm I heard just before going into the Optometry School. No test I had ever taken as a student was as emotionally painful and difficult as this one. A fire alarm was going off inside of me. When I had been a student at UC Berkeley and hadn't prepared for an exam, I could draw on past lectures and readings and compose creative answers to exam questions. With this vision test, there was no maneuvering. Either I could see the cat with a tail and whiskers or I couldn't. I knew what I was supposed to see (the entire cat) but due to my alternating vision, I was well aware that I might only see part of the cat. I was afraid that if I didn't see the whole cat that the doctor and intern would deem me unsuitable for VT. Surprisingly, I could see the complete image with both eyes for a long time and the doctor and resident were surprised that at the age of 31, I could maintain the whole picture for so long. They didn't think that my brain cells had developed enough depth perception capabilities for me to be able to use both eyes.

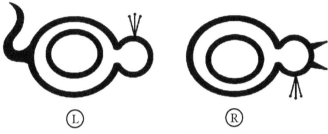

Cat image for the amblyscope. The left eye sees the cat with the left whiskers and with a tail and the right eye sees the cat with the right whiskers and no tail. When both eyes see together, the patient sees the cat with both whiskers and tail.

Image credit: © *Bernell Corporation*

Teary-eyed, I listened to the doctor and resident confirm my appointment for the next week to do another battery of tests.

I left the clinic and walked along the beautiful campus listening to the haunting melody of the Campanile's carillon set of bells. I tried as hard as I could not to erupt crying. I so wanted to know if I was a good candidate for vision therapy or not, but I had to wait. There were so many tests the Binocular Vision Clinic needed to do to analyze my situation that I could not complete them in one visit.

I arrived at the parking lot in Sunnyvale and found a $47 parking ticket on my dashboard. Choosing the environmentally responsible route, I had taken public transportation and doubled my commute time to Berkeley, and all I got was an expensive parking ticket!

When I returned to the clinic, I found out that I did have the capability of doing vision therapy to improve my depth perception. However, the doctor pointed out that I should not have any expectations. I might not be as lucky as "Stereo Sue." Due to the distance to Berkeley and financial concerns, I delayed pursuing the therapy. My health insurance would not cover the costs of VT.

June 2010

I received an email from Sue Barry with the subject line "finxing my gze" with some of the characters looking strange. I didn't recognize Sue Barry's name at first and I wondered if the email was SPAM. I opened it anyway and was pleased to find out that Sue Barry, "Stereo Sue," had published her book, *Fixing My Gaze,* about how she had developed 3D vision in her late 40s by doing developmental vision therapy. (See the Resources section for more information about *Fixing My Gaze.*) I read the book on a flight from New York to San Francisco and couldn't stop crying. Although some of the neurobiological explanations of how Barry's brain worked to create binocular vision were too hard for me to comprehend on my first reading, the sections in her book on how difficult it was to be cross-eyed rang true. As a child, she was in a class for remedial students because she had trouble reading. It is not so uncommon for strabismic kids to be labeled as "slow" even though their main problem is that they see in double and have trouble reading. Barry was most definitely not mentally challenged; she graduated with a PhD in Neurobiology from Princeton University and is a professor of neurobiology. In her studies, she was told that a human brain could never develop the capacity to see in 3D as an adult. Her own testimonies of her awesome journey from 2D to 3D countered the Nobel Prize-winning research of Professors David Hunter Hubel and Thorsten Weisel of Harvard University who showed that adult cats who did not have binocular vision in their early years could not develop binocular vision as adult cats. As a result of their research, medical and optometry schools taught eye doctors that adults lacking 3D vision could never develop binocular vision.

Barry explained in her book that cat brains are different from human brains and are therefore not a reliable source of information about human brain plasticity. The Nobel Prize-winning research on cat amblyopia could not be used as a basis for forming definitive prognoses for adults doing binocular vision therapy.

I was deeply motivated to do VT after reading Barry's book.

One person whom I told about *Fixing My Gaze* and how much I wanted to do vision therapy implored me that he "loves my eyes just the way they are." Although I appreciated the support, this was the problem when I explained my vision to others: because my eyes were cosmetically straight, I first had to convince people that I was actually "cross-eyed" and then I had to explain that what I was seeking was better vision and depth perception, not just more attractive eyes. If all I wanted were prettier eyes, I'd spend money on various color contacts and parade around with blue eyes one day, brown eyes another day, and sometimes let people see my green hazel eyes. Communicating the importance of Dr. Barry's book to those with 3D vision was the first indication that explaining 2D vision and vision therapy was going to be an uphill battle.

CHAPTER TWO

New Year, New World

You know you are in binocular vision therapy when...

1.

You tell people you can see two moons and the only person who doesn't think you're a verified lunatic is your developmental optometrist who asks, "How far apart horizontally and vertically were the two moons? Could you make them come together and be single again?"

2.

Your friend complains he's losing his hair and you tell him, "I can't tell because I see you in double. With two heads, you have a lot more hair than usual!"

3.

Somebody keeps asking you to drive them somewhere at night and you realize you have a good excuse: "Do you really want me to drive you at night? I see double at night. All the streetlights, car lights and other lights either have halos or lots of rays coming out of them in all directions. I have trouble making sense of where to go."

4.

You find yourself staring at napkins because you had never noticed the undulating texture. It looks like an orange peel with all its curves and dips."

5.

At a street crossing, while waiting for the light to turn green, you are distracted from the traffic as you are amazed at the concrete and how unsmooth it looks.

6.

You stare at people you've known for a long time and can't figure out why they look different, until you realize that they have more wrinkles on their face than you had previously noticed! (Hopefully, you don't announce your new finding to the newly-aged person.)

7.

You prefer to go on walks with your friends and family rather than sit with them in front of you across a table because you don't want to see them in double. (Motion cuts down on double vision.)

8.

You finally have an excuse to become a couch potato because you have little energy to do much else.

9.

You have a great excuse to diplomatically excuse yourself from family functions with loud and annoying relatives and family friends: "I can't take the noise. Plus I see some people in double and it drives me crazy."

10.

You can be a kid again and spend lots of time every week staring at Humpty Dumpty, clowns and other children's images and see them in double. You also get to see things that don't exist. You see five dots on the wall, but the doctor has only shone four.

11.

Most importantly, any time you think you are going crazy, you can just blame it on the vision therapy!

12.

You wonder if intermittent double vision is a valid excuse to avoid jury duty.

Socrates:
"Vision is not only what we see, but also what we are prepared to perceive."

Socrates was right: the mind sees what we are ready to perceive. I was ready to see in depth and have my world change but I had no idea the impact this changing world would have on me.

I know I'm searching for something
Something so undefined
That it can only be seen
By the eyes of the blind
I must be lookin' for something
Something sacred I lost
But the river is wide
And it's too hard to cross
Even though I know the river is wide
I walk down every evening and stand on the shore
I try to cross to the opposite side
So I can finally find what I've been looking for

(Billy Joel, *River of Dreams*)

To someone who has seen flat for over three decades, three-dimensional vision is something that is undefined and absolutely unfathomable. It's as though I were traversing my river of 2D to get to the 3D side, having no idea what was on the other side. The song speaks of something sought out and only visible by the eyes of the blind. This is ironic since what I was seeking was actually the norm for more than 95% of the population. To them, I was the one who was "blind"– stereoblind.

2010

Birthday present!

After almost four and a half years of considering the cost of vision therapy (around $100 per session), I decided to pursue the treatment, but I didn't want to travel all the way to Berkeley (an hour each way by car or two or more hours each way via two trains and parking tickets).

I needed to get evaluated by another optometrist located close to me who specialized in this therapy. I asked my friend Savannah for help. Despite having suffered through vision and reading problems her entire life, Savannah still became a high school English teacher. In her 30s, she was afraid she had a brain tumor because her vision became unstable. Once she found out she had **suppression** and **convergence** issues, she did VT to stabilize her vision. Savannah's developmental optometrist recommended a colleague, Dr. K, in my area.

As I was slicing tomatoes on my white cutting board, Dr. K called. I put down the knife and paced along the white squares on the kitchen floor as I described my surgical history and vision. Dr. K said he was one of few optometrists nationwide who had experience doing vision therapy with adult strabismics who had previously undergone surgery. I was happy that he would evaluate me and I decided to make my first appointment with him on my birthday.

Though I didn't need someone inside the office with me while the doctor examined me, I didn't want to go alone. I was worried that if the doctor told me I would not be a candidate for this therapy that I would be distraught, would need moral support, and would not be fit to drive home. I asked my good friend Dilip to drive me.

During the ride, I was anxious about the appointment and preferred to talk about light topics.

The doctor wrote my eye history information by hand and didn't enter anything into a computer. He looked over my vision history and surgery records. I was so used to doctors typing on computers and not writing on paper that I was surprised to see him take physical notes. The doctor seemed to be equally surprised that I had come to see him on my birthday.

"I am giving 3D vision to myself as a birthday present," I said, not realizing that my gift to myself was going to be the most difficult voyage of my life so far.

After performing many tests, he said that I had two conditions, in addition to my astigmatism, amblyopia and strabismus: **anomalous retinal correspondence** and **horror fusionus**. Just the sound of the words *horror fusionus* made it sound like I was in a horror movie! He ended the appointment by telling me that I was a "difficult case, but not impossible." He also said I wouldn't develop full 3D vision but that I could improve my depth perception. Relieved, I left ready to enjoy my rainy birthday.

That evening, I met some friends at an Italian restaurant for my birthday dinner. To take the charge out of my anxiety over my morning eye appointment, I joked about "being a difficult, but not impossible" case with my sister and friends. After dinner, we walked along Santa Clara Street in downtown San Jose to a salsa dance club, to meet more friends.

I had started my new year with the dual goal of gaining stereo-vision and becoming a great salsa dancer. Knowing that I was clumsy, I figured that improving my vision would help my hand-eye coordination and dancing abilities. Little did I know that s dancing and changing my brain and eyes were not activities to be pursued simultaneously.

I started vision therapy with Dr. K the next day and scheduled myself to be in the doctor's office three times a week. Even though Dr. K's office wasn't far from my work or home, I didn't know if I'd feel comfortable driving after my doctor's appointments. I was lucky that my doctor's office was on a major street and if I was desperate, I could take several busses to get home or walk to my sister's office.

Since I was working as a substitute teacher, I was usually done with work around 3:00 or 3:30pm and could make it to the doctor's office in the afternoons. Optimally, it would have been better to come in the morning, before school kids came to the lab afterschool, but that didn't work for my schedule. Other adults doing VT may have to ask for time off of work to make it to the doctor's office during business hours, which could present the challenge of explaining what VT is. I know an engineer in Silicon Valley who had to explain to her boss that she didn't see in 3D and her boss had never heard of amblyopia or binocular vision problems but was supportive of her making up for lost work time during business hours in the evenings or weekends. I am glad I didn't have to make my case in front of anyone to get time off to do VT.

Living in Silicon Valley, where software is constantly being updated from version 1.0 to 2.0 and so forth, friends wanted to know how much better my vision was going to improve. On my birthday visit the doctor was clear that I would not see in full 3D so I was not going to "upgrade" my sight from 2.0 to 3.0 via VT. He couldn't say whether I could get to version 2.5 or even 2.25. I embarked on my birthday journey with much uncertainty but with an adventuresome spirit determined to give my all to make it happen.

Where are the adults?

When I came to the therapy area of the doctor's office, I immediately noticed the absence of adult patients. I was the only patient above three feet (one meter) tall and with a developed voice. Luckily, the chairs were big enough for adults. Most medical doctors who are amblyopia and strabismus specialists are pediatric ophthalmologists. They cater to their child patients by having small chairs and they show cartoons while examining the kids. Many years prior to VT, I had been to see an ophthalmologist specialist at the University of California at San Francisco (UCSF) Medical Center and all of the adult chairs in the waiting room were occupied by the parents. I couldn't fit into the children's chairs and had to stand while admiring the foggy view of the San Francisco Bay from UCSF Medical Center on the Parnassus Avenue hill.

The therapy room at this developmental optometrist's office had computers, a ball hanging from the ceiling, stereoscopic equipment and other unnamed machines. It was like a vision therapy play center. Vision therapists worked with kids on various eye exercises. Not all of the kids had asymmetric eyes; some had reading issues and practiced reading.

To check out VT equipment for homework, I had to fill out and sign a form. Since all of the patients were minors, there was only a signature line for parents or guardians. I had to sign as my own parent or legal guardian!

VT Exercises

The doctor and I sat down on opposite sides of a small table. He explained that we were going to use **polarized glasses** to know if I was using just one eye at a time or both. He introduced one of the main tools I saw in his office: transparencies called **vectograms**, made by the Bernell Corporation.

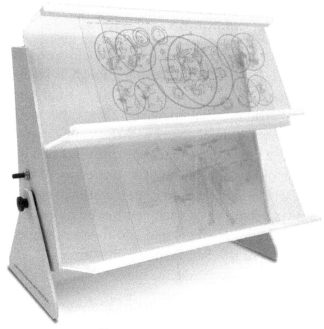

Vectogram in a light box
Image credit: © *Bernell Corporation*

A vectogram is a polarized stereogram consisting of two polarized images at right angles to each other. When viewed through polarizing lenses it presents one image to one eye and another image to the other eye.

There were two quoit vectograms in a light box. Each transparency had a circle on it. The circle looked like it was made of rope. On top of each quoit was a small box with either a horizontal or a vertical line. The vectogram for the left eye had an "L" in a box in the lower left. The right eye vectrogram had the letter "R" in a box in the lower right of the transparency. The "L" and "R" and

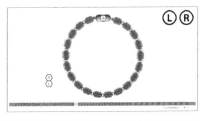

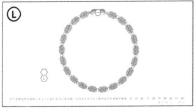

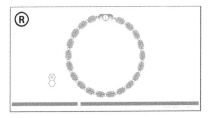

When wearing red-green glasses, the right eye sees the green vectogram and the left eye sees the red vectogram. When both eyes work together, the patient sees the red and green lines cross at the top center of the image and both the "R" and "L" to the left of the image at the bottom.

Image credit: © Bernell Corporation

the horizontal and vertical lines allowed the doctor and patient to know if both eyes were working together. The left eye saw the "L" and the horizontal line in the circle and the right eye saw the "R" and the vertical line in the circle. If the patient saw the horizontal line and vertical line cross in the center of the little box and also saw both the "L" and the "R" simultaneously, then the brain was not suppressing the vision from either eye. The doctor slowly moved the vectograms away from each other and asked me to announce when the image doubled. The goal was to keep the images single for as long as possible and to increase my **divergence** and **convergence** ranges in seeing the image single.

"Don't look directly at the cross at the top. Look in the center of the image and tell me if you can see the lines cross in the periphery of your vision," the doctor said.

As soon as I would move my eyes to look at the cross, it would no longer be in the periphery, but in my central gaze. However, the point was to see if I could fuse in my periphery. It reminded me of the Biblical story of Lot's wife from the Old Testament story of Genesis. When escaping from the town of Sodom, the angels told Lot and his wife not to look back. Lot's wife, curious to see what disaster had struck her town, looked back and turned into a pillar of salt. I had to fight my curiosity and natural inclination to look at the cross at the top of the vectogram. I knew I wouldn't turn into a pillar of salt, but I would be defying the point of the exercise.

Several months later, while watching the Brazil vs. North Korea 2010 World Cup game, I realized a similarity between vision therapy and soccer. The soccer players have to see the ball in front of them and also know how to best pass the ball to their teammates without getting into the hands or feet of their opponents. It's as though the players must have eyes on all sides of their heads and see the center and periphery simultaneously.

Far from being a soccer star, I was struggling to focus on the center and be mindful of the periphery at the same time.

When the doctor walked me out of the session to the waiting room, we passed by a small room with a trampoline.

"Doctor, do I get to do exercises on the trampoline?" I asked.

"No, that's just for kids. You're too tall and you could injure your head if you jump too high and hit the ceiling," he responded.

Peripheral fusion

Another exercise was similar to the quoit vectograms but instead of two circles of the same size, there was a big circle on one transparency and a small circle on the other. The doctor or vision therapist moved them apart. I had to tell them if one of the circles was closer to me. The idea of this exercise was to determine if I could use both eyes to work together and see distance. After a couple of sessions, the doctor was happy to learn that I could indeed tell which image was closer to me than the other, showing that I had peripheral fusion. I didn't see one image popping out but I did see if one image looked slightly closer than the other.

Nose too small for the four lenses

When I graduated to vectograms consisting of more than just circles, I had to put on my regular glasses, Polaroid lenses, red/green glasses and a prism all at the same time to look at double transparencies to see if I could see them in double. Although I was the oldest patient in the room, my nose wasn't big enough for all the lenses and I had to hold the prism with my hand. I didn't know how the kids with even smaller noses handled all of the lenses they had to wear!

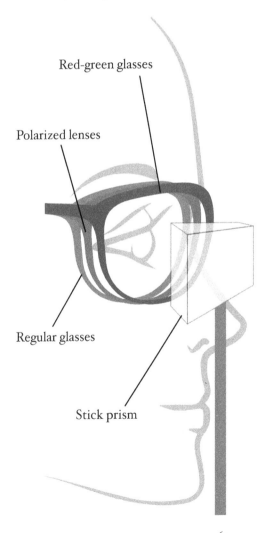

Red-green glasses

Polarized lenses

Regular glasses

Stick prism

A person wearing three lenses (polarized lens, red-green glasses, and prescription glasses) and holding a prism in front of their eyes.

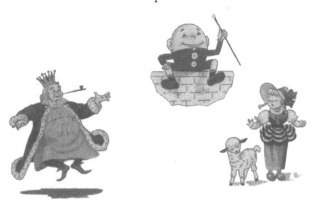

Mother Goose vectogram for the left eye. Image credit: ©Bernell Corporation

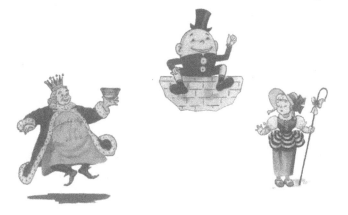

Mother Goose vectogram for the right eye. Image credit: ©Bernell Corporation

Mother Goose rhymes usually evoke fun memories in childhood. The Mother Goose characters in these vectograms were anything but fun. The left eye vectogram shows Old King Cole with his crown and his pipe, Humpty Dumpty at the top with a cane and Little Bo Peep with her sheep. The right eye vectogram has the same king with a bowl in his left hand, Humpty Dumpty has a hat on his head and Little Bo Peep has a cane. The goal was to fuse the left and right images into one.

It was my hardest task yet. I struggled to see what the doctor was showing me. I knew he wanted me to see the complete picture of the king in 3D, with both the bowl using my right eye and the pipe via my left eye. My vision quickly alternated from eye to eye. I could only see the regal man with either a bowl or a pipe, but not both. For someone like me, goal-oriented and practical, it killed me psychologically to not be able to see something that I knew existed. My friend Savannah told me she felt like a paralysis victim when she couldn't make images line up or converge in her VT sessions. Her frustration resonated with me when I did exercises where I couldn't perform obvious tasks.

Clowning around!

I stared at this image of the clown and the boxes while moving either the top or bottom transparency until I saw something double. Then I moved the transparency back until it was single and then repeated the whole process so the optometrist could measure where I saw single and where I saw double. At the bottom of each transparency was a ruler with measurements in **diopters**. When I pulled the images apart from each other, I was testing my divergence ranges to see how far apart my eyes could move and still maintain a single image. Sometimes, my eyes strained as I pulled the images to the outer limits of my range. It was easier to bring the image inwards and test my convergence ranges, but either way, the exercise could still cause headaches and exhaustion.

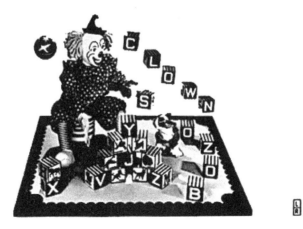

Clown vectogram. Image credit: ©Bernell Corporation

I couldn't be in VT without doing the standard **Brock string** exercise. The Brock string, named after Dr. Frederick W. Brock who was a strabismic optometrist, had three colored balls on it. When looking at one of the balls, the others were supposed to appear in double and that was how I knew if I was using both eyes. The Brock string could quickly strain my eyes. As I got better at the exercises, the doctor altered the length of the Brock string to make it more challenging.

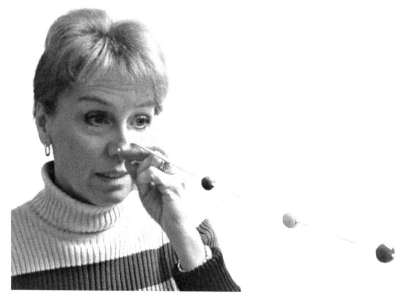

Brock string. Photo credit: © Bernell Corporation

To feel even more like a kid, I got to stare at Frosty the Snowman in a mirror. I taped an image of the Snowman missing a nose or an ear to my bedroom wall. I looked at that image via a mirror with just one eye. The other eye saw the other image of the Snowman missing some other body part. When I used both eyes, then I'd see the Snowman in his entirety. Once he lost an ear or other body part, I knew my brain was shutting off one of my eyes.

Some VT sessions were actually fun, especially when I got to look at a swinging ball through a prism to see the ball in double.

Becoming a kid again
Homework

To make the brain adapt as quickly and effectively as possible, I performed vision therapy exercises at home every day. The doctor would tell me at the end of each session if I had new assignments and informed me if I needed to check out new equipment.

I even took the vision therapy equipment to work and did some exercises during my breaks when no one could see me.

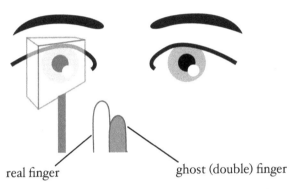

real finger   ghost (double) finger

One of my homework assignments consisted of holding a prism to one eye and looking at objects to see them in double, forcing the eye with the prism in front of the object and the other eye to view simultaneously. I waved my finger around my face, seeing it in single, in duplicate, single, duplicate, and so on. I could not keep the finger double for very long.

Soon after I had started vision therapy, my family and I went out for my sister's birthday. My niece and nephew took the prism and looked at each other and everyone else until they could see them in double. They also had fun making their falafels and kebabs duplicate and then go back to single. My sister was worried the kids would have headaches after seeing things in double with the prisms.

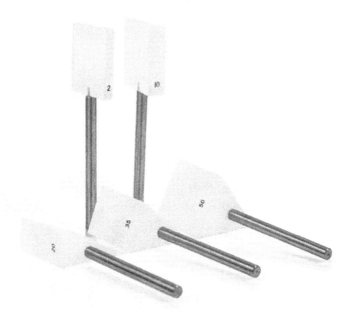

Stick prisms. Photo credit: © Bernell Corporation

Not out of vanity, but out of necessity to work my eye muscles, I had to wear Polaroid glasses and look at myself in the mirror, walking backwards until I could no longer see both of my eyes at the same time. For a moment, I could see both eyes. Then one lens would go black, showing that my brain was no longer processing the vision from that eye. I would approach the mirror again until I saw my two eyes come back in full view. I would walk backwards until one of my eyes became black. My niece and nephew also had fun walking backwards and looking at themselves in the mirror with the Polaroid glasses.

Cartoons for vision therapy homework

My new vision therapy homework was to watch cartoons with my funny prism glasses! I put red and green plastic sheets on the screen while simultaneously wearing my normal glasses, prism glasses, and red-green glasses, amounting to too many lenses to fit on my nose, and I was not Pinocchio! If I could see the entire

TV screen I knew I was using both eyes. Since I saw more depth while in motion, the doctor thought moving targets in animation would be better for me than looking at letters (my normal routine). I welcomed this change! My nephew and niece had to share *Curious George* and other cartoons with their "Auntie with the cuckoo glasses."

When I told this to my friend, he sent me this response:

"Watching cartoons as homework. You are in my childhood paradise, Susanna."

My reply:

"There has to be some benefit for spending so many months wearing prism glasses that make me look like a clown!"

Wearing prism glasses, only at home

These were my new domestic specs. I didn't dare wear them outside of the house over my normal glasses, so I wore them only indoors. The funny glasses made me look like a clown. I felt like I was a child in disguise.

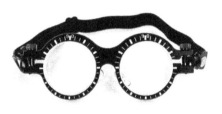

Prism goggles.
Photo credit: © Bernell Corporation

When I first put them on, anything on the corners of the glasses seemed curvy. My sister put them on and saw everything in double. My niece and nephew thought they were so funny looking that they got my sister to take photos of them wearing the glasses. Of course, they wondered why their aunt had to wear glasses that made them see in double. I couldn't explain to them that their aunt didn't see in double with these glasses because she wasn't used to seeing with both eyes.

My world is moving!

One evening, as I was relaxing in my bath tub, I shocked myself when I noticed the tiles of the step leading to the bath as slanted upwards. I'd never noticed that slanting before.

Like a baby discovering the world, I found myself just lying in bed looking around at my room anew, noticing slight changes in objects but being unable to articulate exactly what was different.

I was in constant awe wondering if I was truly seeing things differently or if my mind was expecting changes from the therapy and fooling me into thinking that the bush next to my car was any different from what it had been the day before. I didn't know what to believe.

As an adult in vision therapy, it was mind blowing to see something in single and then have it double and then disappear. The shift from single to double was harder to handle than my childhood "magic power" of moving objects with my eyes, because as an adult, I thought that if I saw something then it must have been real. But if my mind was playing tricks on me and showing me the same object in duplicate and then in single in a matter of seconds, I felt like I was going crazy or living in the funny mirror section of the children's science museum. With time, I learned that if I saw the walls vibrate or the lines on my bathroom tiles move, this was due to the vision therapy.

I went from not seeing in 3D to actually seeing things that were not there. It's as though I came to the movies to see a 3D movie and ended up a character in a science fiction screening instead.

Repeatedly, I'd be sitting somewhere with someone and, out of the corner of my eyes, I would see an inanimate object move on its own. I'd stop the conversation and look at the chair or whatever object I saw move, only to find it in its original position. It was as though I were in a movie where ghosts played tricks on mortals and moved objects around and confused the mortals who couldn't understand why their possessions were located in a new place.

About four months into vision therapy, I went to see my **ophthalmologist** at the Santa Clara Kaiser facility where I had been going for years. I had previously lent him my copy of *Fixing My Gaze* so that he could tell his other strabismic patients about vision therapy. I told him that I had started my therapy and wanted to see if he could perceive any changes in me.

He had me put on red-green glasses and look at some dots he flashed on the wall.

"Doctor, how can I see five dots if there are only four?"

"You are in a confusional state. You are using both eyes, but you are not fusing. Your vertical divergence is disassociated. The signals sent are not integrated from one eye to another."

(I copied this from my notes. He might have also said I was in a non-fusional state instead of a confusional state.)

Non-fusion or confusion. It didn't make a difference. I was seeing things that didn't exist.

What else did I see that was not there? What else was a figment of my confusion, non-fusion or imagination?

In my head

I couldn't remember much about my eye surgery from March 1994 when I got my eye straightened during my senior year of high school. This was one of the most important events in my life and I didn't recall how I felt before or after the surgery. My family couldn't recollect anything either. I didn't think people in high school treated me any differently after my surgery. It was as though my complex about my wandering eye had been all in my head. I emailed my high school friends to see if any of them could remember how I felt before and after surgery. Two of them couldn't recall that my eyes had ever been misaligned. One friend said, "I do remember that the change was dramatic. I never really noticed you had an eye condition—until after you had it corrected."

All that time that I felt like a freak and others didn't think of me that way!

I recalled an episode of the 1980s sitcom *Head of the Class,* when Arvid chose to get a nose job to reduce his nose size. He felt ugly because of his big nose. When he came to school after his surgery, he was shocked that nobody noticed that he "looked better." His big nose complex was all in his head.

After starting VT, when I wore my contacts I had mental flashes of the photo of my eyes in Chapter One, from when I was 13 years old without my glasses, when my eyes were not aligned. Even though my second surgery at age 17 had "cosmetically straightened" my eyes and the VT exercises were straightening my eyes even more, I felt like my eyes had become untethered from their "cosmetically straight" positions when I was despectacled. It was as though I could once again feel the stitches on my eye and the patch I had to wear for one day after the second operation. Before doing VT, I had never evoked the feelings of having stitches or how I looked with stitches after the second surgery. Even though I knew full well that VT had not undone the progress of my two surgeries, the sensation of having noticeably unaligned eyes was a mental illusion due the trauma of the surgeries, VT and memories of how I used to look. My mental image of myself regressed to how I had looked with a lazy eye.

Blu-Ray opened my eyes and made me sad

My Colombian friend Javier wanted to show me what a Blu-Ray movie looked like on his flat screen TV. To say that I was stunned would be an understatement.

While watching the sitcom *How I Met Your Mother*, I noticed more distance between the sidewalk and buildings than I had ever seen before on screen. Also, I noticed the fine lines on people's faces, the texture of their garments and dust flying in the air. I was in awe of the movement on the screen, so much so that I wasn't paying attention to the plot or dialogue, but more to how I saw the images glide from one place to another.

We watched the beginning of the movie *Angels and Demons*. I had never seen such details before, either on screen or off. I had seen *Angels and Demons* a year prior on a flight from Bangkok, Thailand to Doha, Qatar. Of course, the quality of the airplane small screen was lacking, but I had never seen such a contrast of image quality as I had on Javier's Blu-Ray of *Angels and Demons*. If Blu-Ray was the closest technology had come to showing real life, then I had been missing out on a lot of visual details my entire life.

When the actors in the film *The Social Network* and the TV show *How I Met Your Mother* were walking, it was as though they were riding on a moving sidewalk at the airport or riding on a skateboard.

Why was I seeing these details and fluid motion on screen and not in real life?

"Is this how you see in real life? With this much detail?" I asked.

Surprised, Javier responded, "Yes, of course. You mean that you don't see this way?"

"No," I demurred.

Javier explained to me the difference between movie theater screens, regular TVs, DVDs and Blu-Rays, but no matter how much description he provided, I was still in shock.

Actually, I was sad.

I was sad because I had never before been able to imagine what it was that I was missing until I saw the Blu-Ray movie. I could understand the look of bewilderment on the faces of people when I told them I only saw in 2D because I myself was in shock.

Dr. Oliver Sacks stated in his article "Stereo Sue" in *The New Yorker* that explaining 3D vision to someone who is stereoblind is like explaining color to a blind person. It was as though I had been color blind and the Blu-Ray movie gave me the ability to see the rainbow.

Javier and I had previously been speaking in Spanish, but I had to speak in English. It was late and the emotions were so strong that I didn't know if they would come out correctly in another tongue.

"But doesn't it make you happy that you can now appreciate something you've never seen before?" Javier asked.

"I know it seems strange to you that this saddens me, as I should be rejoicing at my newfound ability to see this clearly, but it actually makes me upset," I responded.

The following day, I told this to my friend Jessica and she also thought that I should be happy. I know what the "logical" re-action "should be": happiness with a positive change in vision. But sometimes, the mind does not act logically. Claire, another friend, had told me about, *At First Sight*, a film about a blind man about a blind man who gained sight but was overwhelmed by what he could see. I could understand that feeling. Despite wanting more than anything to see in 3D, the glimpses of depth that I did get sometimes awed and saddened me.

This reminded me of a story my mom told me about when she was living in the former USSR. Her mother's cousin came to visit from Denmark when my mom was a young adult. The visiting aunt said, "You are not sad because you don't know how poorly you live," referring to the dramatic contrast in the standard of living in Soviet Russia with food lines and communal apartments and the material wealth of Scandinavia. Before the Blu-Ray movie, I didn't know to be sad because I had not known what I was missing in my vision.

Seeing life like in a Blu-Ray movie: going from 2D to 3D in real life

The Blu-Ray film became a reference point that I could cite to articulate what I saw to make my observations more understandable for others.

Eight months into vision therapy, objects and people in motion looked different. Hubcaps revolved super fast when I saw cars in motion.

While watching a group of kids play lacrosse after the rain, I was amazed when I saw how the water from the wet grass moved upwards into the air. It looked like a slow-motion sequence from a movie but it was real.

When I saw my friend César playing the guitar, I was in awe at how the guitar strings vibrated. Previously, I would just see the guitar string move from place to place but I wouldn't see the white strings move so slowly up and down. I paid more attention to the vibrating strings than to César's music!

After over a year and a half in VT, I noticed another distinct change in my vision. During the soft light after sunset, my vision was clearer than in the past. It was not that my vision had previously been especially blurry at twilight, but that my vision had suddenly become crisper with VT.

Life in motion seemed more like a Blu-Ray movie. Cars moved more smoothly across the road. When I opened the paper wrapper on my Subway sandwiches, the paper moved differently, in a sharp way.

Since Javier had opened my eyes to Blu-Ray, I went to electronics stores to admire movies on Blu-Ray and HD 3D TVs. I couldn't see any 3D effects on the 3D TVs but the Blu-Ray TVs fascinated me. Like the poor kid in the movies from the 1950s who didn't have a TV at home and stood on the sidewalk, rain or shine, and stared at TVs through the shop window in awe of moving pictures, I went to the electronics stores not with the intention to purchase, but to be amazed by the images with blunt edges that made them stand out more and the smooth movements of people walking on screen.

Luckily, I didn't have to stand outside in the cold and admire the fantastical world of black and white televisions from the sidewalk. I was standing in front of color, HD 3D TVs inside the stores.

When my vision changed such that I could see the crispness and slowness of movement in my daily life without having to stand in the electronics stores and tell the salespeople that I was just "looking," I was ecstatic. I stopped observing a fantastical world on screen and saw it in real life, getting closer to crossing the wide river between 2D and 3D.

> *I walk every evening and stand on the shore*
> *I try to cross to the opposite side*
> *So I can finally find what I have been looking for*
> *(River of Dreams, Billy Joel)*

I go to the HD and 3D TV store

I try to cross to the opposite side

So I can finally find what I have been looking for

Driving the river between 2D and 3D

Around the same time I saw life in motion as smoother, being in my own car while in motion on the highway became more enjoyable. Driving was like in a video game without the oncoming animation.

I was driving to San Francisco on Highway 280 and I felt good about my position in relation to the road. I usually hated driving but Highway 280 with its hills, grazing cows, and lake was pastoral and pleasant. I hadn't been on that road for a while and it felt different. The road unfurled itself below me as I drove. I was acutely aware of the road coming towards me and moving beneath my vehicle, like the images in video games. I hadn't played video games since I was a kid, but I had seen enough race car tracks on video game terminals to make the analogy.

Details: the beauty of flies, dust, and other small things

Mighty flies

Listening to salsa music on my iPod, I am walking near a small farm in Rancho San Antonio and a swarm of flies stops me in my tracks.

The flies move upwards in the sunlight as though they are bubbles in a recently opened bottle of sparkling (carbonated) water or champagne, quickly hopping or jumping from place to place.

I am transfixed. I find a tree stump to sit on and stare in awe. Two women walk by; the one with a stroller uses her free hand to wave the flies away. I want to say to them, "Look at these flies! Isn't it amazing how they move in the air?" But I say nothing.

I sit, waiting for a new swarm of flies to move in between the trees where the sun is shining brightly and where I can clearly see the white flies ascending upwards from the ground.

I am crying because I have never seen flies move in this carbonated way before. I have no one with whom to share this experience. If there were a beautiful deer or bird, I would tell passersby to stop and admire. Or if there were a snake, I would alert others to be careful.

The flies move away. As I walk back to my car, passing the tennis courts, I use the sleeves on my long-sleeved red shirt to dry my eyes.

Driving home, it is hard to keep my eyes steady on the road because of the tears. I am overcome with emotion.

Upon arriving at my driveway, I feel weak in the way one might feel at seeing a newborn baby, being in love or seeing a loved one die.

I am definitely seeing better because I can perceive white flies in the air. The swarms of flies in the sun are my signal to keep going with the therapy despite my hardships. My face is covered in tears. My throat is becoming sore. I know there is a comical element here that my sign from the Almighty that my vision is improving comes via a life-form most people want to avoid.

By the summer of my first year in VT, my visual acuity had improved so much that I could see the small stuff and was amazed. The devil wasn't in the details, the beauty was!

I transformed from a globetrotter marveling at architectural jewels like the Coliseum, pyramids and temples to finding beauty in the minute.

Lady of the Flies: Seeing in more detail

On a visit to San Francisco, I felt like I was amidst a locust storm, similar to the one I saw in the movie *Nowhere in Africa*. However, the storm was of flies and not locusts.

It was an incredibly sunny day and I sat frozen on a park bench. Many tourists came to delight in the Palace of Fine Arts, a remnant of the 1915 Pan American Fair. I was enraptured by the flies near the garbage can. The Palace of Fine Arts was my favorite place in San Francisco but it couldn't seduce me away from the flies. Before starting therapy, I told my friend Matt that even my garbage could look more interesting once I developed depth perception. Instead of finding the garbage can more appealing, the flies congregating near the trash piqued my interest!

Curious to stare at the flies, I went back to a particular creekside trail near where I used to live in Mountain View just to find white flies and stare at them. Having walked by that trail many times, I knew the flies hadn't recently moved in. They had always been there but I had never seen so well to make out their profiles amidst the light.

While walking with my friend Matt in another park, where we had strolled many times, I pointed out my flies.

"Do you see those flies?" I asked.

"Yes, of course I do," Matt said.

"Two years ago, I couldn't see those flies," I said.

Pointing out what I could see helped my friends get a glimpse into my improved acuity. It didn't mean that they grasped what was going on with me but at least I was not as much of a mystery as before. (Referencing clown vectograms and quoits to a binocular person who has never done VT was pointless.)

> **Commenter #3:**
>
> *Actually, mentioning VT to ANYONE (strabismic or not) often seems pointless. My strabismic brothers don't even get it. I tell everyone about what it did for my children and what I hope to achieve anyway :) Thanks so much for sharing!*

I told Elie, another friend who had done VT, about my flies and he jokingly told me I was a cheap date. I didn't need movies or even fancy dinners. I just needed someone to drive me to the park to stare at flies or at dust circulating or rising in a ray of light and I'd be dazzled!

I discovered that egg shells were not always smooth and little water droplets on freshly cut cucumbers were beautiful.

One of the benefits of improving my visual acuity was seeing the stuff other people didn't care about: mold, flies, dust, water droplets on cucumbers and bumps on egg shells. I knew those things weren't going to appear on any pamphlets or websites advertising VT but they made me pause, awe and smile.

Flies and furry flakes, a strabismic's best friends

Flies weren't the only small white things flying in the air that caught my attention.

Some type of tree in Budapest must have been in bloom when I arrived in May 2013 because I saw flurries of white furry things like snowflakes flying around the city. I couldn't help but stop and admire them. I had never noticed them when I had lived in the city. Budapest had many tourist attractions like the Parliament Building, the bathhouses, bridges and Opera House, but the flurries had my rapt attention.

A few days after being in Budapest, I was in Bosnia, walking by the Sarajevo Zoo and again I saw an almost non-stop movement of white flurry things moving in the air above the creek. At first, I thought there must have been some kids blowing lots of bubbles but then I saw that the swarm was of these white flurry things again. It wasn't windy so I didn't know why there were so many, nor did I know from where they were coming. Again, I stood in awe and no one else seemed to care or notice. It was as though it were snowing but the snow was moving horizontally and not vertically.

Missing the big picture

From flurry things to the sand, details stood out.

While lying on the beach by the Seaside sand dunes near Monterey, California staring at the sand, there appeared to be more black space between the grains of sand. Could this be the greater depth to which I was aspiring? I looked at the waves, the dunes, the view of Monterey and everything looked the same as before. Only the sand was different. In vision therapy, the doctor told me not to worry about the small details I saw changing in the vectograms. But it was precisely the details that I saw change; the big picture stayed the same.

My car seat, towel, sand and grooves on the highway cement appeared to be more defined. Looking at the deeper grooves on the road was not a good idea while driving. I wondered if, as my vision improved, I would realize how many potholes or other problems there were with roads I had previously seen as perfectly flat and normal.

On another weekend getaway to the coast, I sat on the famous white sand beach in Carmel in a sundress. Despite the clear sky and magnificent sun, the wind made it cold. When I got up to leave the beautiful cold white sand, I looked at the goose bumps on my skin. I couldn't believe how huge the bumps were. I couldn't tell if they seemed to be big because my sense of depth had improved or if I really was so cold that the goose bumps had become so large!

The next day, I was eating a burrito at a Mexican restaurant, and found myself staring at the napkins. I had never seen napkins before with the detailed undulating texture like that of an orange peel. Perhaps I had never seen this particular brand of restaurant napkins before, but I had eaten at the same restaurant a year prior. I definitely hadn't stared at the napkins in awe of their deep design the previous year. I couldn't imagine that there was such a variety of restaurant napkins that I had never used this particular kind previously.

Months later, another detail popped out at me. I looked up at the overhang coming from the roof on my parents' house and noticed the texture on the pink painted wood. I had never noticed the texture before, although I had probably seen it many times.

However, it would be strange for me to say that I saw more clearly now than before VT because my vision had never seemed unclear or shallow. I saw what I saw. It wasn't blurry. To say that my vision was clearer was like saying that what I had seen previously was unclear. But it hadn't been.

Steam, fumes, mist and mini rainbows

Whether it was sand or napkins, small, almost invisible things captivated me.

Usually, when I took a shower in the cold, I turned on the mini heater in the bathroom. One day, I didn't turn on the heater. When I finished my shower, I opened the shower door. Water dripping down my body, I stood in reverence of the steam by the window. I didn't even put on my towel. I blew on the mist to see the water droplets change direction. I marveled at the steam rising from my body in waves.

Steam was not a new addition to my life, having seen it many times, especially when opening a pot of boiling potatoes. The difference was that I always had my glasses on in the kitchen. I didn't have any corrective lenses on during my morning shower, proving that my visual acuity had improved during VT because I had never before seen steam in such clarity with my naked eyes.

The best view of the steam and mist was by the window because the sunlight coming through made the steam easier to see. The steam and mist moved in various waves through the sun rays. I could see individual tiny water droplets, like those rising from the mist of a waterfall.

After that instance, I didn't turn on the heater in the bathroom anymore, even if it was cold. I wanted to enjoy looking at the steam for as long as possible. If I turned on the heater, I would see less mist because there would be less of a temperature contrast between the water and air.

Smoke and sprinklers

What was even more surprising than steam and flies was when something from across the street would grab my attention, like cigarette smoke and sprinklers.

I abhor tobacco and the malodorous fumes from cigarettes and cigars. I used to live in the former Yugoslavia, where "No Smoking" signs were a strange decoration in buildings and ignored by all smokers, including government officials whose jobs it was to post the signs. I used to refer to bars and cafés in Sarajevo as "overcrowded ashtrays" because the stench from the omnipresent smokers was so heavy that my hair and clothes would stink after a few minutes of being in these venues. For cigarette smoke to stop me in my tracks, it had to be an extraordinary event. One day, when walking in San Francisco, close to the Chinatown gates, I was about to cross the street to enter Chinatown when I saw an Asian man across the street smoking. Usually, the sight of someone inhaling lung cancer would not make me take notice, but this time I missed the green light to traverse the street to watch the smoke from this man's cigarette. I could see huge—big for just one small cigarette—fumes all around this man's hand. It was as though he had a fire burning in his fingers and the smoke from the fire was easy to see and formed dense, wide and large clouds around him. Usually, smoke would rise from a cigarette in a couple thin fumes but this was much larger.

I would also stop to see mist rising above my neighbor's sprinklers. If the sun was shining just right, I could see the mist forming smaller droplets from the sprinkler and rising upwards. Once, my neighbor from across the street saw me staring at his sprinklers and asked me if there was something wrong. I wasn't comfortable telling him about my VT so I just told him that I was seeing a mini rainbow forming. I really did see a faint rainbow, but I had seen those before and they were easier to spot because of the many different colors. But when I could see small transparent drops of water from across the street, I knew my vision was becoming sharper because the target, the mist, was not only tiny, it was also transparent and harder to see than a red color in a mini rainbow.

Dust: my omnipresent friend

Even dust was captivating. I was a chaperone for my nephew's class trip to San Juan Bautista, a Spanish mission and historical site. After about an hour in the noisy yellow school bus, one of the nine-year-old boys threw up and his vomit spilled onto the corridor of the bus. When we returned to the bus after the visit, there was a light smell from the vomit still in the bus. My nephew was playing with my nails and then fell asleep on my lap. Instead of being annoyed at the noise of the chatting kids and vomit smell, I was fascinated by all of the flying dust alit by the shining sun coming through the window. The dust was moving in all different directions, like snow in the wind. Sometimes it was just suspended in the air.

Often, I stared at the dust coming in through a sunray in the window or in a dusty car. Friends would apologize for their cars being dirty, but I quietly appreciated the flying dust moving in the light.

Birds and the bees and I look at trees

Seeing nature in a new way gave me a verdant alternative to the dust.

I was staring at trees, rose bushes and other shrubs! I walked slowly, admiring how the tree branches, flower petals, leaves and ferns seemed to be reaching out to me as I approached.

I was taking the bus (even when I didn't know the destination of the bus) just to see trees in motion. It was cool to see the trees closest to me move past me while the images in the distance stayed still. Apparently, when I explained this to 3D friends, my new sight was normal to them. I couldn't recall how things looked before, but they were certainly different. Dr. K said that I was seeing the trees in motion on the street as I should have been. I noticed this arboreal motion effect while driving on a street near my house. It felt as though the trees were a canopy moving above me and opening up as I drove in the middle of them. It was hard to stay focused on the road because it was so beautiful to see the trees and feel the road move under me. I realized that driving this way was unsafe and that I would either have to ask someone to drive me around or I'd have to take the bus. I didn't want to talk or listen to music; I just wanted to admire the trees. Finding someone to drive me around in silence seemed unlikely. I moved around the bus to see which seats afforded me the best views.

The optometrist explained this phenomenon with the trees as **motion parallax**, a type of depth perception cue in which objects that were closer to me appeared to move faster than objects that were further away. My binocular vision was activated while I was in motion; no surprise there as I was a traveler.

I liked to walk a lot in silence and admire trees. It felt as though tree branches were just sticking out at me. When the wind blew, the full branches looked like some underwater plant moving in the water.

This was a very isolating experience because I hadn't found anyone locally who shared my fascination for staring at trees. I walked around with my head pointed upwards to admire the arboreal splendor. I probably looked like I was on drugs or was delirious or an accident waiting to happen. I could have easily tripped and fallen since I wasn't paying attention to the sidewalk, just the trees above.

I felt like an alien from another planet, happy to see trees for the first time and admire roses. It was a good thing many of my neighbors had beautiful rose bushes that moved towards me as I approached and that there was a rose garden not far from my home.

I was also noticing spider webs. When walking into my dad's shed, I was taken aback by all the spider webs and how complex they were. I saw them at the park, especially on bushes. During one walk in the park, I stopped, picked up a stick and unraveled the webs on the bushes and plants. Who else, besides young kids, would be having fun breaking apart spider webs? One day, I witnessed a spider making a web. I was amazed by the spider I saw moving in the air, suspended by nothing.

One of the advantages of spending so much time admiring nature was that I became acutely aware of the seasons and the early autumn leaves. Even before our turn to fall, I noticed autumnal hues of orange and red on trees. I mentioned this to a friend who lived in foggy San Francisco, commuted on a tree-less highway and worked in an office. She had no idea that the trees were already showing signs of change. Evidently, she didn't spend much time admiring the beauty of trees.

When I took the plunge to do vision therapy, I knew my vision was going to change. However, I had no idea that small things like steam, flies and dust were going to rock my world and literally make me stand in reverence with water dripping from my body and not care about my plans and tasks for the day or drying myself off. Slowly, I was appreciating being in awe of discovering things that few others appreciate. I had this little world that was all my own. One person's garbage (dust and flies) was another person's treasure. These small details made me enjoy seeing the world for the first time, over and over again.

It was heartwarming to receive this comment from a reader who understood about relishing the slowness of life and the beauty of trees.

> *Commenter #1 says:*
>
> *I too spend a lot of time walking around at lunchtime in a park looking at the trees and the long walkways and the space between the people and branches, which until vision therapy, I had never noticed. I catch myself stopping and staring at the oddest things.*

Negotiating with my vision

The best way to describe my changing vision was that it was like negotiating between what I saw and what I knew was real. Looking at things and registering what they really were was time-consuming.

Visual distortions

After three months of vision therapy, I had a succession of incidents several days in a row that caused me great confusion as many things moved around me. The extra time it took to make sense of the distortions took me away from my activities.

I felt as though my eyes were not stable. While walking on the sidewalk, I saw the diagonal lines moving along with me as I walked. They had never moved before and had always stayed in the same place as I went past them.

When I explained this to the optometrist, he said that my eyes were alternating between **esotropia** and **exotropia** quite quickly, giving me the feeling that I was not stable because things moved around.

With esotropia, a person uses only one eye to look at an object while the other eye turns inward.

With exotropia, a person uses only one eye to look at an object while the other eye turns outward.

Exotropia is the opposite of esotropia.

Once, when I was looking out the gym window, it seemed as though the license plate of the car parked by the window was inside the gym, not outside. I had to look closely and it still appeared distorted. But I knew that the car was definitely outside the gym and not inside.

The day after my gym incident, while driving on the highway, I looked in my rear view mirror and the cars behind me seemed to be curved upwards. They should have been in a semi-straight line behind me. I blinked, looked ahead of me and then checked again in the mirror. The cars had returned to their normal position.

The doctor said that these optical distortions were actually a good sign because they meant that my brain was momentarily fusing; however, the brain shut off quickly because it was overwhelmed with too much information.

Seeing two full moons: What is real?

I stood in my aunt's backyard at my cousin's birthday and looked at the moon. I saw the moon in single. Then I worked my magic by doing something with my eyes I wasn't conscious of and I got to see two moons! The second moon wasn't quite the same size as the "real" one, it was more of an oblong shape and it moved around. I could keep it double for a long time.

As a result of my double lunar novelty, the doctor gave me a new homework assignment: to look at a piece of white paper with one letter in black until I saw it in double. When the letter doubled, I had to use a prism on my right eye to make it single. He explained that the contrast of the light of the bright moon on the night sky might explain why I could see the moon in double.

This experience made me wonder how one could know what really exists if one can tell oneself to see in single or double. My entire notion of what was real came under the microscope. The only reason I knew there was just one moon and not two was because for my whole life, I had only seen one moon. While other planets have multiple moons, the Earth has only one. But what if someone had diplopia all their life and lived somewhere in the jungle where there was no optometric care? (Though for all I knew, the local shamans may have had their own cures for double vision that didn't involve prisms and Brock strings.) Would that person, seeing in double intermittently their entire

real doorknob   phantom doorknob

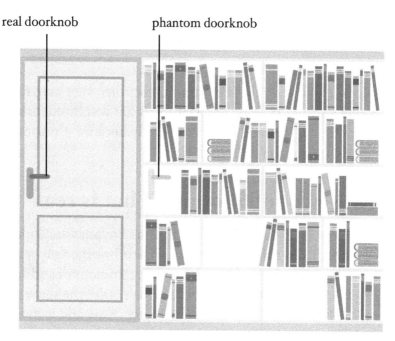

Juxtaposed doorknob on bookshelf

life, think that there were two moons? Would they have an explanation for why they sometimes saw one moon and on other days, two moons? So much of what we take as a given, our reality, is what we see. But when my brain was showing me something different from what I knew to be real, I questioned my reality.

This constant questioning was not only distracting but cumbersome. If I saw my doorknob appear on top of my Spanish-English dictionary sitting on my bookshelf, I had to remind myself that my doorknob had not, on its own, unattached itself from my door and flown to be suspended in midair in front of the dictionary.

Tan the strabismic way!

The strabismic alternative to a spray-on tan was another mental exercise in negotiating with my reality.

For a quick tan, some people buy "spray-on" tan formulas, while others go to tanning salons and burn themselves in tanning beds. I found a safe way to 'tan.' One caveat: the only person who will recognize the tan has to have **alternating vision**.

I was talking to my former landlords in their living room in Sarajevo and suddenly, Mustafa's face became darker. I stopped paying attention to what he was saying in Bosnian about Ottoman history and got distracted by his face. He looked like he had just spent a week on the coast under the sun. But he hadn't gone anywhere in the split second from when his face appeared paler until the moment he looked tan. I hadn't moved anywhere. Ash hadn't fallen from the ceiling and landed on his face.

My brain was using my left eye instead of my right eye. The window was on my right side. When my left eye was leading, there was less light reflected on Mustafa's face from the window and he looked tanner. My brain was focused on the vision from my left eye and suppressed my right eye.

Imagine talking to someone and seeing their face change from white to tan and trying to pay attention to what they are saying in another language. It's difficult not to get distracted. My brain had suppressed vision from one of my eyes most of my life so that I would not be distracted by quick movements and changes in color. It was good that the VT had made my brain use both eyes but the result was that I felt confused. The goal was for my brain to fuse the images from both eyes so that I wouldn't have such strange situations viewing a person's face changing hues.

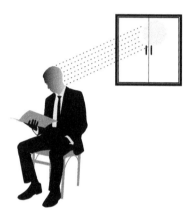

When I look at the person in the chair with my right eye, the face looks lighter because of the sun on the right.

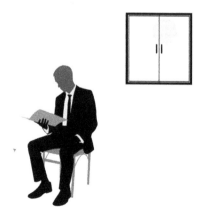

When I look at the man with my left eye and I don't see the sun rays on this right, his face is darker

Commenter #9:

My first childhood memory that my alternate way of seeing different colors is described here http://leavingflatland. wordpress.com/about-lynda/. I believe the pink vs. blue coloration I was seeing was due to the warm light coming in from the window to my right vs. the cool light I was seeing from the left shadow side of my face. I was swiveling back and forth in a dining room chair, looking at the white Formica table in front of me: pink, blue, pink, blue ... of course my mother had no clue what I was talking about!

My first sight of 3D, pretty cool!

After 11 months in VT, I saw in 3D once with 3D glasses while watching a 3D image on the computer at the optometrist's office.

I'd seen this scene many times before on the computer screen: a Dunlop brand soccer ball moved from the bottom of the screen to the top of the screen with a backdrop of some men on the soccer field in different colored jerseys. In the past, I had seen the ball double at some point. This time, the soccer ball went out of the screen. It appeared as though it were halfway between me and the computer screen. I even showed the doctor where I perceived I could catch it. He was happy that I was finally seeing a 3D image! I thought it was really cool.

P.S. I never saw the image again or anything else pop out of the screen.

My Sue Barry "raindrop" moment

One of the signature scenes in Sue Barry's book, *Fixing My Gaze*, was when she spent her lunch hour sitting in the snow marveling at the dimensions of and space between snowflakes on a winter day in Massachusetts. Forgetting to buy lunch, she stared at the snow, in awe. On another occasion, after a snowfall, she lay down on the ground to look at fallen tree branches. A colleague of hers walked by and asked her what she was doing lying in the cold looking at branches. She tried to explain the amazing image before her, but her colleague couldn't understand a grown woman's newfound amazement at fallen tree branches, something Barry must have seen every winter of her life.

Snow is rare in Silicon Valley, California, where I resided, so I wasn't anticipating a Sue Barry snowflake moment. But it happened. For me it was rain drops.

I walked out of the Cupertino library on a rainy evening *sans* umbrella towards the parking lot. The headlights of a car in the pick-up lane made me freeze. The bright light shone through the rain. The rain drops fell onto the ground and repelled from the cement in a V shape. My hair was getting wet. I held my book bag close to my chest to prevent it from getting soaked. Cold, wet, and anxious to get home, I stood on the walkway motionless, staring at the raindrops. I must have looked strange to anyone scurrying to get to their car before getting drenched but I didn't care because I'd never seen rain drops form a V when boomeranging off of the cement. "This must be my Sue Barry snowflake moment," I thought to myself. The car drove away and then I couldn't see the magnificent rain drops so clearly anymore. This was not my only time seeing rain illuminated at night by headlights. However, I perceived more distance between rain drops and could see separate drops.

Other days, I'd catch myself staring out the window at falling rain. Before VT, I couldn't always tell if it was raining or not as

I couldn't see the rain drops clearly, especially if it was a light rain or only sprinkling. When I was looking through windows that had an overhang above, the rain was at least a foot (33cm) away, not right next to the window. At that distance, it was hard to see transparent rain drops. I often relied on other cues to determine if it was raining: the sound of water hitting the gutters, the light sound of the falling rain, wet sidewalks, smell of new rain and glistening grass and plants. If I were to tell my friends, "Wow, I can finally see the rain!" I would have felt silly because I had not lived in a desert all my life. No one would understand how special it was for me to know it was raining just by seeing the rain and not by using other clues.

Commenter #2 says:

Wow! That is exciting and marvelous!

Commenter #10 says:

You are no longer a One-Eyed Princess!

Thanks for sharing your wonderful raindrop story!

Rain looks like snow

I was in Sarajevo to do research for the documentary *Saved by Language*, which I was co-producing. It rained for seven out of my eight days there. I had many an opportunity to look at rain and appreciate it. The rain was so white that it looked almost like light snow. To my misfortune, with my cloth shoes, I wasn't prepared for the rain. One very rainy night, I was waiting for my friend Ivan to come and meet me in front of the Central Bank. He was running late and I stood below an overhang to keep from getting totally wet, staring at the falling rain illuminated by the light in the tall lamppost. I was smiling and appreciating the distance between the rain drops although my feet were cold and wet.

SNOW!!! In more depth

Three years into VT and halfway across the world, I saw snow in more depth and it was incredible! Unlike Sue Barry, I wasn't so dazzled by being in a 3D dance with snow, but I was amazed at how I could see the snowflakes individually and clearly. (I'd lived in places with snow and was no stranger to winter flakes.)

Dressed in my blue wool coat that made me look like I had just stepped out of the *Dr. Zhivago* film set, I stood on the main street of the Armenian city of Gyumri. My mind was distracted from the terrible destruction of the city by the 1988 earthquake. The front lights of a car at night illuminated the snow falling down like a fireworks display, each flake quickly moving at a different angle.

During the day, the sight of the snow reminded me of the opening scene of the movie *Hugo*, which I had seen in 2D. In the film, there were either snowflakes or dust falling into the train station and each flake approached the screen, as though the flakes were coming towards me as I was sitting in my red velvet movie theatre seat. On the Armenian street in daylight, I could see both the snow closest to me and the snow a few meters (more than six feet) away and across the street, all at once. I loved looking at the flakes of snow on the fur at the end of my winter coat. The droplets of water from the snowflakes rested on the strands of fur, like in some nature photography show where the water droplets on flower petals are super clear and large.

All I could hope for was for it to snow again so I could just sit and stare. I couldn't truly explain how I had seen snow before. It hadn't been as clear or well defined. And the snow definitely hadn't come towards me like a cascade of fireworks.

Commenter #13 says:

Congratulations!! You've just unlocked the Santa Barry's Badge! ;-)
#binocularenvy

Commenter #9 says:

This is wonder-FULL. I hope you get to see more snow in more and more depth each time. Every once in a while, I see texture in detail both near and a little farther away and have a moment of discovery, and enjoy this multi-level way of seeing. Let's carry on!

Commenter's blog about VT:
http://leavingflatland.wordpress.com/about-lynda

Close to Ten: slowing down

It's no secret that I am a *musicophile*, a lover of music. My friend Gautam recommended a song, *Close to Ten* by Tina Dico. When I heard it, I felt an automatic connection as it reflected how I felt about my eyes and getting to 3D.

I placed in bold the lyrics that stood out to me. On the right side, my comments are in italics.

Original	My comments
There are faces, there are smiles, so many teeth, too many arms and legs	*There are so many facial features in double, people appear in double.*
And eyes and flashing buttons all around me	*The walls vibrate loudly.*
I'm a-watching, I'm a-breathing, I'm a-pushing, I'm a-wishing	
That these walls would not be talking quite so loudly	
I have lost it once before I've pulled myself up from the floor	*Vision therapy is often too much for my brain to take at any one time.*
And I am looking for a reason to stay standing	*I had to pull myself off the dance floor after falling because I got dizzy from the movement and lights.*
But sometimes it's just too much or not enough or something else	
It's so much bigger than my head, it's too demanding	

Original	My comments
I'm gonna close my eyes And when I open them again Everything will make sense to me then	*I can't close my eyes throughout VT or else I won't make any progress. But I do want what I see to make sense. When my eyes change, I'll see life anew.*
I have met so many people, we've exchanged so many words We've said it all and we've said nothing but it's changed us In the wild, entangled gardens of our insecurities We lose our heads into each other's hidden pitfalls **Sometimes the fastest way to get there is to go slow** **And sometimes if you wanna hold on you got to let go**	*I've been slowing down my life to accommodate my eyes and brain. I have to let go of my old life.* *I've exchanged many words about VT with others, only to be hurt by their silence, leading to more of my insecurities.*

Tous les dimanches du monde: All the Sundays in the world

In March 2011, there was a noticeable slowness about me, partially caused by my lack of a car due to a recent car accident that had left me without wheels for three months. Beyond my transportation problems, I just moved slowly. I am usually a fast walker, but that March I often strolled slowly, as though I had nowhere to be and no time constraints. It was as though every day was a Sunday and everything around me moved slowly!

There was a French movie starring Gerard Depardieu's son, Guillaume Depardieu, called *Tous les matins du monde* (*All the mornings of the world*). Although my life doesn't replicate the movie's plot set in 17th century France, the title of the film reflected how I felt. March was a month of all Sundays. It felt like there were fewer cars on the road. I walked around and stared at trees and at my neighbors' homes and flowers as though I had never seen them before.

My life was moving slowly, but it wasn't without its compensations. It was as though by looking at the world anew, I was a visitor from another planet whose sense of time was much slower. However, my go-getter self was not keen on the slowness of my VT and how everything else in my life seemed to be moving at a snail's pace. Media pieces I was interviewed for months prior, were not published until months later, people took a long time to return my calls and emails, etc. Incidentally, I also sold more books (*Language is Music* and *Travel Happy, Budget Low*) that month even though I hadn't done much promotion.

Humbling return to Berkeley
June 2013

Not only did I have to change my rhythm of living, I also had to step back into my past and feel like a student again at UC Berkeley, but this time I wasn't a student with homework. My new assignments at UC Berkeley were about changing my brain.

In June 2013, I switched from my local eye doctor to the UC Berkeley Binocular Vision Clinic. I felt like I had reached a plateau with my previous doctor and I was ready for a slightly different approach. Since I had taken a few months off from VT before recommencing at Berkeley, my eyes and brain were rusty.

I would get super tired and get headaches after VT at Berkeley. Sometimes, I would take a nap on the grass somewhere on campus to recover. One time, I was awakened by a dog licking me! Despite being no friend of canines, I could still see the humor in being so tired that only a curious dog could wake me up!

I returned to Berkeley not as a student but as a patient, and I rediscovered the campus as someone with a renewed interest in seeing the world. During my breaks, students scurried quickly from classes and discussed upcoming tests. I sat on the grass by Strawberry Creek and admired the squirrels hopping around. I especially enjoyed watching their mouths move quickly as they ate acorns, details that I had never noticed during my tenure as a student. When I wasn't in a rush to meet someone or go back to the BART (train) station, I walked slowly around the campus, taking in the architecture and the details on the buildings that I hadn't noticed as a student. I even found a special parking lot reserved for Nobel Laureates that I hadn't known existed!

I went to the Morrison Reading Room at the Bancroft Library to sit in the leather chairs and listen to opera music on the CDs I borrowed from the receptionist. Even during the digital music age, when so much music can be purchased at the touch of a button on a screen, I still took delight in borrowing a recording of Puccini's *Turandot*, relaxing in the comfortable leather chair, closing my eyes and melting into "Non Piangere Liù" and other arias. Sometimes, I'd look at the chandeliers, peruse the old records or smile at the students dozing and occasionally snoring. As a patient in need of ocular recuperation after doctor's visits or during breaks between sessions in the lab, I enjoyed being a visitor, savoring the beauty and energy of the campus.

It was difficult getting to Berkeley on a weekly basis because I had to drive in rush hour traffic for 30-45 minutes to the Fremont BART station. When there was an accident or a lot of rain, it was impossible to make it to the station on time and find a parking spot. On those days, I had to drive through heavy morning traffic to Berkeley and arrived utterly exhausted. The clinic was very popular, and it could take two to three months to reschedule appointments, so I never wanted to miss an appointment, even if I was tired or sick.

Fatigued or not, I had to do my best to train my eyes to work together. The resident in binocular vision therapy often assigned me to work with the cheiroscope. While fighting to draw a simple triangle using the cheiroscope, with one eye seeing the image of the triangle reflected by a mirror and the other eye seeing my pen on the paper as I traced the triangle, the image kept moving. My eyes were shifting. I had to wait until I could get my eyes to bring the triangle back to its original location.

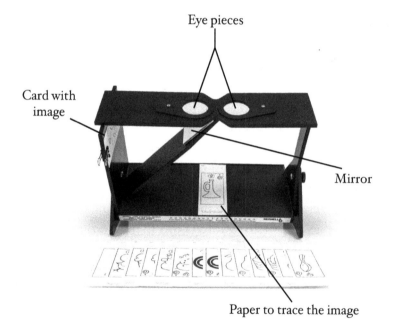

With the cheiroscope in this position, the left eye sees the image on the card while the right eye sees the blank piece of paper on which the patient traces the image seen with the left eye, forcing the brain to merge the image in the left eye and the paper in the right eye. When the patient flips the cheiroscope around, the right eye sees the card with the image and the left eye sees the paper.

Image credit: ©Bernell Corporation

The doctor had me do some drawings using the cheiroscope with my left eye seeing the reflection of the picture and my right (dominant) eye working to bring what it saw of my hand holding my pencil on the paper.

Imagine tracing the image you see reflected on the mirror. However, you have to use both eyes to be able to see the reflection on the mirror, on the left, and what you are drawing on the paper on the right side of the cheiroscope. If you can see with both eyes, this is not hard. If you alternate from one eye to the other, this can be excruciatingly difficult.

The triangle kept moving!

This was like in the movie *Hunger Games,* when the couple was succeeding at surviving in the forest but the rulers of the game decided to make it harder and added a rainstorm and animals chasing the couple. Just when I thought I had the lines of the reflected triangle matched with the one I was drawing, they separated. The scene reminded me of the quote my friend Liz had on the wallpaper in her bathroom: "Just when you think you can make ends meet, somebody moves the ends." That was exactly how I felt when drawing my triangle or the other geometric figures which moved. Someone had moved the ends. However, that someone was my brain!

Drawing this triangle on the university campus was one of the most humbling experiences of my life. It felt like getting a PhD in Physics, a subject I hadn't studied since high school and one at which I was an average student, would have been easier than drawing this triangle. Tears were coming out of my eyes as I struggled to draw something even preschoolers could draw and I couldn't. I had graduated early with honors from UC Berkeley at the age of 20, only to return in my 30s at a pre-preschool level. I was devastated at how low my simple drawing skills were.

After almost eight months in the UC Berkeley clinic, I moved to be a research patient in the Optometry School, where Drs. Dennis Levi and Roger Li were running experiments on adult with amblyopia using computer exercises and video games to test if those exercises helped to improve **stereopsis**. I had to come for about 16 hours of testing over a couple of weeks to see if I even qualified for the study. I left the lab with any mixture of fatigue, headaches, nausea and hunger.

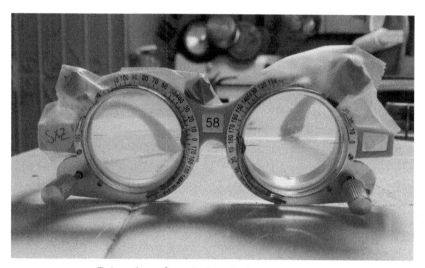

Prism glasses from the Levi Lab at UC Berkeley.

When Dr. Li examined me, he chose his words carefully when he said he was "cautiously optimistic." I could imagine the machinations in his brain as he silently pondered my case. Having been in this situation before, observing doctors thinking deeply about my complex case, I knew better than to talk and ask questions. I reciprocated his silence and waited for him to speak. I wasn't expecting a miracle cure, nor anyone being overly enthusiastic to take me on as a research participant given my surgical history and difficulties with VT and its side effects. At this point, I had been doing VT for four years, and despite my progress, I had yet to develop depth perception. I had spent a lot of money on VT and was recovering from the impact of all of the side effects (discussed in the next chapter). I was desperate. I was elated when Dr. Li accepted me into the study. An added bonus to being a research participant was that I got paid a small amount for my hours in the lab—a major improvement from spending lots of money on being a VT patient.

Being in the lab gave me much more than vision exercises. I listened to Dr. Li explain aspects of binocular vision to his lab assistants, which helped me get a deeper knowledge of what was going on with me and others. I finally had the community I had been longing for ever since I had started VT. In the lab, I met other adults and kids with my same condition. There was a Latin American lady who flew in monthly from Miami to do exercises in the lab. Like me, she didn't understand why she had so much trouble driving until her adulthood. She came to our lab for the *"ultima esperanza"* (last hope).

I could ask for advice, trade stories and feel understood. I had people with whom to laugh at our situations. The sounds of adults and children playing video games made my experience more pleasurable. Once, while playing a video game, I was paired with a 10-year-old. He quickly tired of my hesitations and unfamiliarity with the game and grabbed the controller from my hand! After that, we both played the video games alone. Nonetheless, the atmosphere was always congenial and supportive.

I had to spend over four years in VT until I ended up in a windowless Berkeley lab with little ventilation, many computers, a dirty floor, scientific papers with ribbons that the lab researchers had published, and post-it notes with various research participants' prescriptions hanging above the case of prisms to finally have a place where I felt comfortable. This lab was within a seven-minute walk of the International House residence hall where I had resided for two years as an undergraduate student at UC Berkeley! If only I had known about my condition when

I was a student, I could have done the therapy then. It would have been even better if I had known about this as a child.

VT rebirth

Before I had become a research participant at UC Berkeley, I desperately longed for people with whom to share my experiences who could appreciate what I was seeing. In the absence of companion VT travellers in my immediate surroundings, I gravitated more and more to my sister's kids because they were nearby and found my VT exercises "cool" because the exercises made them see in double. They were ages three and five when I started my VT journey, and I felt like I was growing up with them. Even though they didn't stare at flying dust with me for as long as I did, they at least acknowledged its presence when I pointed out the waves of dust I marvelled at when the sun shone through the windows.

With my social life limited to daylight hours unless I could get a ride to social events, I spent more and more time with my niece and nephew. One week, I spent several nights watching *Sesame Street* in English, Russian and Spanish with them, when they were ages four and six. Instead of dating people my age, I had a DVD date with the Cookie Monster.

My niece and nephew liked doing my homework with me and taking down my measurements. I called them my coaches. They called themselves my "butt kickers" because if I didn't do well, they had to kick my butt to try harder! I got stickers when I did a good job and beat my scores from before! Not only were they my VT task masters, but the closest people I had to companions.

When they were eight and ten years old, I invited them and my mom and sister to visit me in the lab in Berkeley to see the equipment I was using and the video games. They were so excited to step into my world. The kids ran to me to give me hugs by the water fountain between Boalt Law School and the Phoebe A.

Hearst Museum of Anthropology. Natalie was jumping around the fountain into my arms and I was afraid she would fall on the ground.

Despite the lab not having a candy bowl, the kids enjoyed the lab, even the boring computer exercise. They mostly liked the video game, even though my sister got a headache as soon as she tried the game! I was glad my family experienced the exercises, even if they could not understand the complexity of the changes in my brain.

At the clinic and the lab, I was always surrounded by children and I felt like I was becoming a child again, seeing the world anew.

I was much better at perceiving depth while I was either in motion or I was seeing something, like dust, moving. In Barry's book, she cited the research paper, "Preservation of Position and Motion Stereopsis in Strabismic Subjects" by Japanese researchers Hiroshi Kiraoji and Kesiuke Toyama, where "Their experiments demonstrate that strabismic individuals who flunk the standard stereopsis tests used in the eye doctor's office may be able to see in 3D when they look at large or moving targets when looking in their peripheral visual fields." This explains how I had some coarse stereopsis when in motion.

Friends often wondered what kept me going in VT despite my many frustrations. Besides my determination, the small glimpses of progress that I saw were my little breakthroughs. Each person doing VT will find their own source of motivation and inspiration.

Latin dance night, St. Stephens Pub on Castro Street in Mountain View, California

I have just danced five salsa songs and I feel like I am going to faint. The multicolored lights above me seem to be multiplying.

It's too hot inside. Suddenly, the dance club feels crowded. I can't focus on my salsa dance steps. I keep saying, "Lo siento. I am sorry" to my dance partners.

I want to walk outside and get away from the noise and the lights, but I'm wearing just a sleeveless dress. I pick up my light sweater. I wave to my friend, Gladys, who is getting a drink at the bar.

"I'm going outside for some fresh air," I tell Gladys.

I step outside of the bar and pass the bouncer sitting on his stool, only to be met by some men wearing black leather jackets speaking in Spanish and smoking by the door. I move away from the smokers and stand on the sidewalk looking at the long line of people in front of the gelato store. I slowly breathe in the tobacco-less air and look around.

What is going on with me?

I have been to crowded dance clubs before.

Why is today so hard for me?

Everything seems so overwhelming. I don't feel like I am myself anymore.

Even on the sidewalk, the music from the dance club is loud and clear. I can't escape being bothered by the volume. I sing along to the new salsa hit, "Yo no sé mañana" ("I don't know about tomorrow") by Luis Enrique.

Being in the fresh air, I regain some clarity and energy and return to the dance club. I struggle to make sense of the noise, people, colors and lights. I don't know what's going on with me but I don't feel right.

Like the lyrics in the song, "I don't know about tomorrow. This life is a roulette that spins without stopping," I don't know if I'll have the energy tomorrow to be myself. My life is spinning when I dance, objects are moving, and other times, I am seeing in double. I don't know if tomorrow will be better or worse. My life is out of my hands.

– CHAPTER THREE –

Side Effects

Timeline of major side effects

January 2010: major fatigue, double vision, major reduction in social life, noise sensitivity started one to two weeks after the start of VT

Summer 2010: seeing a double moon, inability to drive at night

Fall 2010: intensification of double vision and language confusion

Summer 2012: double vision while driving with the wrong prism glasses prescription

Vision therapy affects patients in different ways. I've met only one person who had no side effects from doing vision exercises to see in 3D. One woman I know could no longer ride in a bus, car or other moving transportation with her eyes open because seeing things moving around her made her nauseous and dizzy. She also couldn't read any more because her double vision was so bad that her mother and husband had to read her graduate school textbooks to her. Like me, she became super-sensitive to noise and could hear the hum of a water heater or fan from over 20 feet away (over 6 meters). Side effects may vary. Some people become super reactive to smells and get nauseated.

When we activate parts of our brains which have been dormant all of our lives, our whole brain goes on overdrive and we become aware of much more than what we previously saw, felt, smelled and heard.

My already keen hearing became even more acute, and I developed aversions to certain people's voices and accents which I had previously tolerated despite not liking them. I had to quickly exit places and social situations where the volume level was so high that I struggled to hear people's individual voices, much less what was in my own head. At home, I had to wear the noise cancellation headphones I had bought to wear on airplanes to diminish the sounds of my neighbor's construction projects, the television, and other people's conversations. I stopped going to some social outings because I knew I could no longer stand certain people's loud voices. I even ceased celebrating my own birthday in the company of others because the confusion of too many people talking at once drove me crazy. In order to survive, I became a hermit.

Starting to lose my mind

There were times during sessions and homework when I needed to close my eyes and take a deep breath. I was getting tired seeing the images on the vectograms appear, double, disappear and go back and forth from one state to another.

By the 5th VT session, I began to feel like I was truly losing both my coordination and my mind. After therapy, I rushed to the gym to attend my Zumba class. Lost, I stood watching the instructor and other students dance around to some Latin American music. Though I'd only taken this class twice before, I knew it wasn't hard. I couldn't understand why I was moving my arms and legs at the wrong time. Frustrated, I left the class early and came home to prepare for a date. I turned on the water to draw a bath and waited for it to heat up, frustrated at how cold it was. Then I looked and saw that I had indeed turned on the cold water instead of the hot water. I knew something was going wrong. After my bath, I laid down on my mattress and closed my eyes, hoping to regain my composure. Luckily, I made it through my date without falling, hitting anyone, knocking over tea cups or tripping.

On another day, I had concentrated so hard at the doctor's office to make an image go double that I was in the same frame of mind when I went to a bookstore cafe to wait for my friend Luis. I looked out at the bookshelves and could tell that my eyes and brain were trying to see them in double. Though I knew very well that I was no longer in the doctor's office and not supposed to see the Barnes and Nobles shelves in duplicate, my brain was involuntarily trying to do so. When I was about to see in double, it felt like when you are about to sneeze and your hand is ready to move to cover your nose but you don't sneeze. When looking at an object, I sensed something was about to quickly change in my vision, but like with the expected sneeze, nothing happened. When Luis arrived and I told him how I was feeling, he offered to drive me home. I appreciated the offer, but decided to go alone. Driving home, I was conscious that my brain was still trying to see in double.

I stopped at a Mexican deli and ordered food for that night and my lunch the next day. I came home to find my housemates on their knees cleaning up the garage after the water heater had exploded and flooded the garage. I explained that I had had a rough day at the doctor's office and I went to my room and ate on the floor. Embarrassed that I couldn't help them clean up, I didn't want my housemates to see me eating while they were doing the dirty work in the garage. I ate quickly and collapsed on my bed, sleeping more than 10 hours.

Fatigue

I am driving to Berkeley to see off a friend moving to Boston. After 20 minutes in the car, I stop for a coffee. I am exhausted even though I had slept well and didn't have to wake up early. Nonetheless, my brain is on overdrive from the vision therapy and the pre-vernal spring heat.

I switch lanes to exit the highway and am stuck in bumper-to-bumper traffic on a highly popular freeway exit. I make it to the first shopping area and all the signs are in Chinese. I don't even like coffee, but when I am tired and have a headache, coffee will bring me to a lucid state and eliminate the throbbing in my head.

I walk into a Vietnamese Pho restaurant and order Vietnamese iced coffee.

"This coffee is very strong. Did you know that?" the waitress asks.

"Oh, yes, I know this coffee very well. When I was in Hanoi in 2007, I had a strong Vietnamese coffee with condensed milk that made me feel like I had electric currents going through my body."

A mild electric shock is needed to restart my system.

I take off my glasses while waiting for the young Vietnamese woman to bring my sugary caffeine. With my head bent towards the table, I hold my head in my hands, massaging my lobes and temples with my thumbs.

The cold overly-sweet brown liquid drips down my throat in slow sips. I continue massaging my head. I get back on the road and let the heat dissolve the ice so I can drink the rest of my coffee on the highway.

Driving to Berkeley, I feel awake again. My headache dissipates.

My friend and I were going to visit my favorite piano bar in Oakland, but by the time I navigate through Berkeley's rush hour street traffic, I have neither the desire nor the energy to do karaoke to the tunes of Sinatra and Porter. Pizza, some wine, chocolate and fun conversation are all I could fit into my head.

This drain on my energy lasted throughout my time in VT, with highs and lows. The most difficult time was my first year.

Fatigue had a major impact on my life as I never knew when either my visual suppression would break down, causing me to see double, or when I would be exhausted. My social life suffered tremendously as a result.

I took my fatigue and sudden onset of headaches and disorientation as signs that my brain was working differently.

When I spoke to my ophthalmologist and optometrist about the ups and downs in my energy levels and my sudden need to sleep, they explained that my brain was overwhelmed with new sensory input from both of my eyes that the only way to get me to stop using my eyes, and brain, was to make me feel so tired that I would have to sleep. Even on days when I had little going on, I felt tired.

My brain had been suppressing vision from one of my eyes all of my life to avoid my seeing in double. I alternated from one eye to another, but I mostly saw with my right eye as I was right eye dominant. Breaking down this suppression was a monumental task!

Rewiring my brain made me rewire who I had always known myself to be since I was a child: energetic, not needing caffeine. It was rough for me to get used to the VT sapping my energy.

Instead of going out dancing or doing something fun, I stayed at home reading or doing something mellow. I was not the type to be in bed by 9:30 pm, but my body had other plans for me. I was fighting the physical manifestations of these changes. I knew I needed to rest, but I didn't want to. The first year was the worst in terms of my fatigue as I'd often sleep 10-12 hours a night. After the first year, I slept normally (around 7-8 hours a night). However, the fatigue would come back when I did new exercises.

Coffee!

On my birthday, the same day I commenced my VT journey, my friend César had given me a Starbucks gift card. There was something both César and I didn't know about each other at the time: we were both amblyopes. As my onset of major fatigue started, I called César from the car as I was driving to excuse myself from an event he had planned.

"I can't attend tonight's event. I am doing this eye therapy to straighten my eyes and improve my vision and it's making me really tired," I said.

"Do you have amblyopia?" César asked.

"You know what amblyopia is?" I said, surprised to hear the word from someone other than my eye doctor.

"Yes, I have it too. I did that therapy and now I can play tennis," César said.

César had gone through VT 20 years prior and had to walk around with an eye patch like a pirate. He knew what the side effects were and understood about my fatigue.

I used up the gift card very quickly as I often needed a coffee. My doctor's office being next to a Starbucks was of great utility. I needed caffeine to keep me awake for VT and for my drive home afterwards and to stave off the vision therapy-invoked headaches. I even had to re-learn how to use a coffee grinder and coffeemaker.

Life in double

Javier calls me and asks to meet in person to tell me something important. Since I can't drive at night, I ask him to come over.

He tells me about his shock at finding out that his new girlfriend is married and that her husband won't grant her a divorce.

His face is serious and worried. His nose and mouth appear in duplicate. I fidget in my chair. I move my eyes from his face to my food, just to break up the diplopia temporarily and not make it obvious to Javier that I am having a problem.

I fight my desire to laugh and smile because Javier looks funny to me with his double facial features. He is afraid of the consequences of his paramour and I can't bear to see him suffer more by my giggling. When I can't keep myself from seeing his face go back and forth from single to double, I suggest we go for a walk in the neighborhood. I know that when walking, I will see less in double. Motion breaks up the brain's ability to create double images because of the speed at which images change.

As we walk, I am not seeing in double, but I am wearing my glasses with a temporary prism sticker affixed to one lens to help me converge the images from each eye. The lines on the sidewalk move along with me as we walk. The sidewalk isn't always flat; sometimes, due to prior earthquakes or growing tree roots, it is elevated in some places. The only way I can walk without falling is by looking at the ground. Even with the varying heights of the sidewalk and seeing moving lines, I am still better off than seeing Javier's facial features duplicate.

When I watched the movie *What the Bleep Do We Know?* about quantum physics, I didn't quite understand the concept of something being present in two places at once because I saw the film before VT. It wasn't until I saw the movie the second time while in VT, that I really thought that something being present in two places could be true. Since I started to occasionally see in double, I could attest to the fact that an object could indeed appear to be in two places at once.

When I saw my walls vibrating, I often thought of the movie *What the Bleep Do We Know!?* because I felt as though I had microscopic vision and could see the atoms of my walls moving around. Ironically, my mom had worked at the Stanford atom smasher facility in the 1980s. I had no idea what the machine did at the time because I was a kid and didn't know anything about physics. It was ironic that, as an adult, I felt like my eyes were atom smashers.

The only other person I knew who had spoken about double vision was my father. When his diabetes was very bad, he had double vision issues and couldn't work. But in his case, he took some eye drops and after a while, his double vision went away. He thought that with just a couple drops in my eyes, my double vision would disappear. I had to explain to him that my diplopia was actually caused by something quite different from his eye trouble.

Binasal blockers

I asked my developmental optometrist if there was any way to stabilize my side effects, as my energy levels were volatile. I had gone to my regular doctor to make sure I didn't have anemia or some other problem that could have been causing the fatigue. My blood tests were all fine, so I deduced that my vision therapy was causing my fatigue.

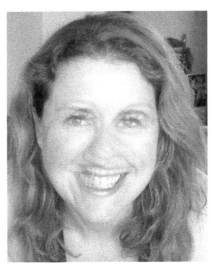

This is how I would look in double with duplicate eyes, eyebrows, nose, mouth and teeth.

I often saw things moving. In mid-sentence, I'd stop because I was sure that I had just seen an inanimate object move, only to realize my brain was playing tricks on me and probably switching the image I saw from one eye to the other.

The doctor suggested I bring in an old pair of glasses for him to tape up to block the vision from one of my eyes so that I wouldn't see in double. I thought he was going to put black tape on my specs and that I would look like a total freak show. Luckily, when I brought him the glasses, he measured in millimeters how much clear tape he would put on the part of my lenses closest to my nose. Though better than black tape, the clear tape was very obvious. I looked like the classic picture of a nerd with

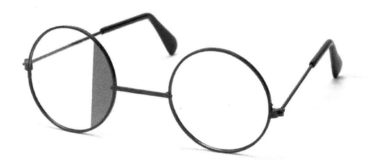

Glasses with tape to block double vision

taped up glasses — not the ideal image for a single woman! The doctor told me I didn't have to wear them *all the time* if I wanted to save myself embarrassment. The night I put on the glasses with the binasal tape, I had a throbbing headache. I don't know if it was because of the binasal tape or if it was due to the vision exercises. But the moving and vibrating objects ceased to catch me off guard. My world stayed stable, at least visually.

The next day, I went to my Brazilian Portuguese conversation group. I didn't want to introduce myself as the taped glasses woman *em português*, so I wore my contact lenses. When I got home and gazed at the vibrating full moon, I saw two full moons.

When I came back to the doctor and told him about my double moon, he chuckled. Then he took the glasses with the tape away and had me do some exercises with my other, untaped, spectacles. He came back with a new look for my lenses. I now had clear nail polish where the tape used to be. The nail polish was less noticeable than the tape. My friends laughed when I told them I had nail polish on my glasses and not on my finger or toe nails. At that point, I really didn't care. If the nail polish could block the sight of incessantly moving objects and keep me sane, that was fine with me.

Seeing double on the highway

Not only was the moon in duplicate with my contact lenses, but many streetlights at night were doubled as well. This was particularly difficult one summer day when I wore my contacts for two interviews I had on Spanish language TV in San Francisco about my language book, *El idioma es música*. I most certainly did not want to appear on television wearing glasses with nail polish! Dr. K cautioned against wearing contacts and I only wore them on special occasions a few times a year. I took out the contacts in between the interviews, but not after the last interview. As I drove home on Highway 280, the reflectors on the left side of my lane were appearing in duplicate. But the reflectors' newfound twins were in a curved formation along the left side of my lane. I had to pay close attention to stay in my lane and not cause an accident. It was so bad that I exited the highway and found a lit Trader Joe's parking lot where I could easily take out my contacts and put on my glasses in my car.

Later my doctor explained that the contrast between the dark night and the lights from cars and streetlights could cause the double vision.

Prism: even the doctor's head is in double

The doctor ordered prism stickers to put on my glasses to see how they would affect my vision. Before ordering new glasses with prisms, he first wanted to see if the stickers would help me fuse. I didn't want to expect a miracle from the stickers, but I was anxious. As a young girl, I collected stickers of ponies, Strawberry Shortcake and other items. I had to laugh when my medical intervention ranged from nail polish to stickers.

When the optometrist put the prism sticker on my glasses, instead of fusing, I intermittently saw the doctor with two heads. It's hard for most people not going through binocular vision therapy to understand why seeing the eye doctor with two heads was a sign of progress, but it was. I was using both of my eyes. The prism sticker reduced my vertical divergence. Even though the doctor's head was in duplicate, his "two heads" were closer together that they had been without the prism sticker.

Better in motion

While in Monterey, on the Californian coast, I rented a bike for four hours and cycled part of 17 Mile Drive, from Cannery Row to the Lone Cypress, all through Pebble Beach, and back. It was gorgeous to ride along the coast. As I switched from my glasses with the prism sticker on the right lens and binasal blockers to my photochromic glasses that got dark in the sun, my brain had to continually re-interpret what I was seeing. With my prism glasses, everything appeared to move when I shifted my head because of the lines on the prism sticker. When I had the photochromic lenses on, images were darker because the lenses adjusted to sunlight and became dark. I would sometimes look outside of my glasses to see what the real colors of the coast were.

The glasses with the sticker and nail polish didn't completely solve my doubling issue. Since those stickered glasses looked weird, I didn't want to wear them and explain to people why I had a sticker and nail polish on my glasses, so I wore my photochromic lenses in most social situations.

The doctor said to switch between the two pairs to exercise my brain. Sometimes, in the middle of an activity, I changed specs to keep my brain alert and working.

I had always been a person in motion. It was easier for me to be in motion than to sit still because I maintained my sanity and saw less in double. Oddly, this seemed counterintuitive because all vision therapy exercises at the optometrist's office required me to sit or stand still and concentrate.

Double Trouble

I was in Miami to promote my book, *El idioma es música*, on foreign language learning in the Spanish language press. I didn't think I was nervous, but as I was waiting for my interview on CNN, I saw the TV screen in double. All the images on the screen were in double. I began feeling nervous. Luckily, when it was my turn to speak on live international TV, I no longer saw in double and my nerves were calmed. However, when there was a delay in the audio and visual signals and the earpiece was falling out of my ear, I had to hide my frustration. To make the situation even more difficult, the TV interviewers asked me to sing a song in Spanish. After a few verses of the famous *Cielito lindo*, I forgot the lyrics on live TV!

A few days after the CNN interview, I was at my friend Montserrat's concert and I saw her with two heads. Usually when I had seen people with two heads, the second head was near the real head. But this time, Montserrat's second head was near her chest.

A few days later, I didn't seem tired at all, but while saying goodbye to my friend Daniel in a parking lot, he also appeared with two heads, with the second one around his waist.

When I reported the sightings of the duplicate heads, the doctor asked me where my friends were standing in relation to me and I said that they were to the right of me. Montserrat was about 10 feet (3 meters) away and Daniel was 5 feet (1.5 meters) away when their extra heads appeared. The doctor told me that my right eye was moving vertically when I looked to the right, explaining why my friends' second heads appeared vertically displaced.

From stickers to real prisms

Two and a half years into VT, the optometrist prescribed glasses with prisms since I had been frequently complaining of double vision and moving objects. He had to modify the amount of prism to adjust to my changing vision.

A common issue optometrists have to deal with in patients who have prism glasses is the issue of prism adapting. My eyes got used to the 10 diopters of vertical prism in my glasses. Instead of having my two eyes stabilize at the same vertical location, my eyes compensated for the prism by moving upwards to their pre-prism level. So the doctor reduced my vertical prism from 10 to 4 prism diopters.

When I got my new prism glasses with less vertical prism, floors appeared to angle upwards and some spaces seemed bigger than before. I knew my living room hadn't become larger but it looked that way. I often found myself staring at floors or looking at corridors to see if the surface would angle upwards. Every day with my new glasses was like seeing things in the funny mirror section of the museum because objects looked bigger, wider or more slanted than before. I was my own walking prism entertainment system! While my brain worked to adapt to all of the new ways I was seeing, I still had to maintain a professional life and not show others how I was more interested in staring at the floor than listening to their serious conversations.

Driving in double

I had to stop driving at night, which meant that I couldn't be out late unless someone drove me. Each and every headlight, brake light and street light grew to be about six to seven times wider than normal. Traffic lights doubled. When I got prism glasses, my intermittent doubling was reduced. I saw fewer objects moving abruptly but the prism glasses made driving more complicated: the left divider lane doubled at a 20° angle. With subsequent changes to my prism glasses, this issue was reduced.

Language Confusion

While trying to make sense of the world, I underwent debilitating verbal processing problems due to VT.

I had been promoting language learning by doing videos and TV interviews in various languages. I was interviewed on the BBC, CNN and other media outlets about how to learn languages efficiently with music, TV, movies, radio, and other media. I was supervising the translation of my book, *Language is Music,* into Spanish. My timing could not have been worse. As the translator sent me his translated versions of my book, I was fighting to stay awake because I was sleeping 10-12 hours a night. I had to drink a lot of coffee and force myself to compare his translation to my original. I had been passionate about this topic for so long and I wanted this book to be successful in Spanish, but it was hard for me to stay awake. It had nothing to do with the quality of the translation; I trusted the translator. It had to do with the fatigue. But I plowed through it and finished.

As I got more and more into my therapy, it wasn't just that it was hard for me to stay awake; it was hard for me to speak coherently in English. My language confusion was not just with foreign languages; I even had trouble with my strongest languages. I am a native Russian speaker and I had lived in the US for so many years that my English was far better than my Russian. In the middle of a phrase, I would stop because I couldn't think of a word. Suddenly the word would come to me, but only in Russian. Instead of saying the word "sign" in English, I remembered the word first in Russian, "вывеска" (viveeska) and then I said the word "vivacious" in English because the Russian and English words sounded similar. I knew that the phonetic cognate in English did not mean what I wanted to say, but I was stuck. I felt like a stroke victim who, in the middle of a sentence, couldn't find the word that they needed. I struggled with this and I felt frustrated and embarrassed because I was young and should not have had this type of mental confusion.

I went to see a neurologist because of my language problems. The doctor told me that although he had never had a patient like me, it made sense that I might have some verbal processing problems because I was overstimulated with information. He said that he sometimes confused Chinese and Spanish and that there was nothing I could do to keep my languages straight. He prescribed magnesium and riboflavin supplements and recommended silence, tai-chi, yoga, meditation, massages and hot baths. He suggested I avoid caffeine, chocolate, cheese and cured meats. However, sometimes without caffeine, I was too tired to focus because of VT, so I couldn't avoid caffeine completely.

It was confirmed: silence was golden!

Pressure of TV

My local Spanish TV station in San Francisco offered me my own segment of a morning news show, where I taught English to Spanish speakers using songs. I carefully crafted my scripts, picked songs, and memorized the songs and lessons that I was going to deliver. I wrote everything out in Spanish so that it would appear on the teleprompter. The first filming day was on a holiday, Presidents' Day, and all the downtown parking lots near the TV studio were closed. I finally found a place to park several long blocks away from the TV station. As I was quickly walking down Howard Street, I saw one of the signs on the street go double. It was rare for me to see in double while in motion and I was worried that my vision was breaking down. I thought, "Oh, no. I can't tape eight segments in Spanish with double vision. This will be terrible." As I continued to walk, the double vision went away. I got to the TV station, had a cup of tea in the break room and looked out at the Financial District and Bay Bridge over the San Francisco Bay. I caught my breath and reviewed my scripts. I was a bit anxious about the teleprompter because I had never used a professional teleprompter before. Reading text and speaking it simultaneously was difficult, especially in a foreign language, so I was under even more pressure to perform. Luckily, my vision didn't go double while I was reading the teleprompter.

Knowing I had this problem with confusing my languages and not being able to find words, I had to prepare even more to make sure I did things correctly so that it wouldn't appear to the public that I was struggling. I would have ruined my own reputation making public mistakes in mixing up languages. How could somebody who talks about the ease of language learning and how multilingualism improves brain function, stumble on TV and mix up her languages?

When I went back to Miami I stayed at my friend Montserrat's place while I had more interviews on Spanish-language TV and on CNN. Montserrat invited me to a French party. I knew I couldn't be in a French-speaking environment because the next day I had an interview in Spanish on TV and I would be doing the interview in my contact lenses instead of my glasses. I had to do everything I could to prepare myself mentally, including cordoning myself off from other linguistic influences. I needed to get enough rest so that my brain would be completely focused. Before VT, I would have had no problem going to a French party one night and speaking in Spanish the next day. However, I knew that I couldn't count on my brain because it was overtaxed with stabilizing my vision. Being overwhelmed with many sensory inputs, my multilingualism was actually making my life more difficult. It was a good thing that I did not attend the French party because the next day, Montserrat was driving me to another *CNN en Español* interview and I accidentally said something to her in Italian rather than in Spanish! Adding French to the mix would have put my Spanish interview in jeopardy!

Going cuckoo in Baku

Being in the oil-rich capital of Baku in Azerbaijan made it hard for me to speak in English!

Azerbaijan was part of the former Soviet Union for many years and Russian was a required language in the country. Most Azerbaijanis still spoke the language, often seamlessly switching from their native Turkic tongue to Russian.

At one restaurant, I said to my fellow colleague, "I wonder if they have a place for unemployed people" instead of saying "I wonder if there's a non-smoking section." My brain and my mouth were not on the same linguistic page at all.

It got so bad that I went to see an Azeri neurologist who ordered me to get a CT scan of my brain, and an electroencephalogram (EEG) where the technician put a bunch of electrodes on my head to test my brain waves. The CT was fine, but the EEG showed spasms and nervousness. The neurologist told me to take a mild tranquilizer, stay away from coffee and take Vinpocetine, a synthetic compound derived from vincamine, a substance found naturally in the leaves of the lesser periwinkle plant (*Vinca minor*). The Vinpocetine was supposed to increase blood circulation in the brain. The neurologist thought that the headaches and fatigue could be due to not enough blood circulation in the brain going to the binocular vision cells that I was re-awakening with my vision therapy. She also prescribed fish oil, gingko biloba, Vitamin E complex and blueberry extract to improve brain alertness.

I knew I had jumps in energy, but I was not so psychologically unstable that I needed a medical tranquilizer! I decided against buying any of the medicines in Baku and waited until I got home. I did stay away from all caffeine to calm myself to deal with my newfound language mess.

Having travelled to other parts of the former USSR with groups of foreigners with whom I had to speak in English, this was my first time with such a language traffic jam in my head. I knew this linguistic confusion was a result of the VT because all of the other factors in my life had remained the same.

Unfortunately, these problems didn't stop by the Caspian Sea. Three years into VT, my language confusion got to be so bad that I had complained to the optometrist that I was becoming more clumsy than usual and had trouble coordinating my hands, eyes and speaking abilities. The doctor gave me an exercise where I had to read letters from a chart to the beat of a metronome and move my arms and legs around at the same time. It was like a medical version of the *Hokey Pokey* dance that I had learned in elementary school. When I did the exercise with my eight-year old nephew, he beat me every time. My coordination skills were less than that of an elementary school student. Just like my not being able to draw a triangle with the cheiroscope in Berkeley, I felt like my coordination skills had regressed to those of a toddler. I was mortified.

Two years after going to Azerbaijan, I returned to the Caucasus to be an election observer in Armenia. I did my metronome exercises quietly in my hotel room, covering the metronome with a towel or blanket to muffle the sound. It needed to be just audible to me but not loud enough for my neighbors to hear it.

I didn't want a repeat of the language confusion I had experienced in Azerbaijan. While staying in Armenia, I was reading the Russian translation of the book *Yeni Hayat* (*New Life*) by the Nobel Prize winning Turkish novelist, Orhan Pamuk. I had started reading the book a few months prior in Indonesia and had no problems with the Russian. Once I heard Armenian-accented Russian spoken by Armenians in Armenia, every time I read the Turkish novel, all I could hear was the book read in my head in Russian with an Armenian accent! The accent was driving me crazy because I couldn't even speak Russian with an Armenian accent, yet my brain was manifesting it upon reading this novel. I had to stop reading the book. This was my third trip to Armenia and I had been going back to former Soviet republics every year or two and this was the first time I had heard a foreign accent in Russian in my head!

Who needs disco lights when your vision is changing at night?

Adding to my language confusion were the optical distortions I experienced. There was no need for a disco ball for me to see lights moving around and changing color; all I needed was to have my vision in flux.

While having a drink at a sidewalk cafe with a friend, each time I moved my head, I saw the streetlights move very quickly as though I were driving past them in a rapid swoop. But I wasn't moving quickly, I was moving my head normally. My one beer could not have made me delirious. My brain was causing the confusion.

The following day, I was inside a cafe for a concert and I could see the lighted sign from a business across the street so closely that it looked like the sign was on the cafe window, but it was across the street. I had to concentrate to make sure that the sign was indeed across the street.

Driving home from the cafe, I saw the green light change to a crimson while transitioning to yellow. Although I wanted to, I couldn't stop midway in the intersection to examine the color. I had never seen the color change so quickly and been able to appreciate the range of colors the stoplight went through to get to yellow. It was as if time had slowed down and I could perceive the green becoming yellow while passing through a red-orange phase.

Cracked glasses

A major factor derailing my progress in VT was the period when I was unknowingly wearing cracked glasses.

Before going to Azerbaijan, I noticed that I was having a lot of trouble driving at night because I saw halos around lights and huge light rays going 10 feet (around 3.3 meters) up and around street lights, car lights, and traffic signals. I could drive only very short distances at night because I would see many lights everywhere. Each light was a starburst with rays going in all directions like a drawing of the sun. Unable to drive, I was stuck at home and felt very annoyed.

In Azerbaijan, although I wasn't behind the wheel, the lights were driving me absolutely crazy. While in the car with my driver, interpreter and election observation partner at night, I had to close my eyes to pay attention to what my partner was saying. The fast moving lights of the moving cars on the opposite side of the freeway were bothering me so much that I could not focus on his words. Another time, I was inside a room with no natural lighting, trying to listen to my former Dutch election observation partner from a prior mission in Ukraine. Due to the overhead lights, I was fighting with all my might just to concentrate on the Dutchman's face and what he was saying. If I moved my head just a bit, rays of lights from the light bulbs above me moved quickly and distracted me. Using the excuse of needing fresh air, I left the room to escape the lights. I didn't want to tell him about my vision problems.

After returning from Baku, I made an appointment with Dr. K and explained my problems with the lights in Baku and not being able to speak in English.

The optometrist couldn't see a connection to the lights problems and my brain since I had the same problem with the lights with one eye closed or both eyes open. I told him that with contacts, I didn't have the starburst problem at night. He was puzzled. He asked to see my glasses and then put them under a microscope.

The culprit was not my brain but my glasses! The anti-reflective coating on my glasses was cracked and creating the odd refractions of light that made me see starbursts and long rays of light at night. The optometrist told me to wear my other glasses that were not cracked. It had taken over a month to figure out the cause of my problem!

I came home, found a pair of glasses I had bought at Costco six years prior and voila! I could drive at night again! I went to the coast for the weekend and was ecstatic. I had my freedom back!

Ever since my change of specs, I had a lot of energy, no night driving problems and no need for caffeine.

Commenter #4 says:

Wow, that's funny that it took that long (weeks?) for the doctors to figure out that it was just your glasses. But I'm glad they figured it out!

I responded:

Yes I was amazed that it took so long for people to figure it out. When I went to the neuro-ophthalmologist in San Francisco, his fellow in neuro-ophthalmology mentioned that my glasses were scratched but didn't connect the scratches to the starburst. Sometimes the best solutions are the most simple!

Partial house arrest: doctor's orders

"Doctor, I need help. Two weeks ago, while whirling around to a merengue song, the room was spinning with me. It was like the scenes in movies when people are super drunk and are rotating, seeing all the lights going around them really fast. But I was completely sober. I was a twirling dervish but there was no mysticism or spiritual purpose to the revolving disco ball and lights above me. I just needed to stay on beat and follow the lead. To avoid getting confused, I fixed my gaze intensely on my dance partner.

I wanted to stay longer, but after an hour and twenty minutes, I had to go.

I went to a Carnival ball last weekend with friends and was wearing a mask. I danced the waltz, mazurka, polka, tango and other dances and had a lot of fun. During the first dance, I was waltzing and the room was moving too fast around me as I turned. Later, the mazurka was so fast I felt like I was literally being swept off my feet by the great leader with whom I was dancing. Halfway through the evening, the motion and twirling around got to be too much and I sat down.

Another time when I had gone out dancing, I was confused by the disco lights, and I fell. Nobody helped me get up," I explained, exasperated.

"Susanna, you need to dance less. Maybe only one time a week. You need to take things slower. Your brain is really busy," the doctor replied.

"How about places with lots of people? I leave shopping malls quickly and get flustered in other places with lots of people," I explained.

"If you feel overstimulated, you should stay away."

For an active person like myself, being told that I was best off to avoid places with lots of people, noise and different lights was about the same as being put on house arrest. It was hard to entertain myself without being around music and people. I had to cut down on meeting with friends because I had a narrow bandwidth and had less patience and interest in listening. Not aware of this at the time, I was in the denial stage of the grieving process. It was too hard to admit that the therapy I was doing for my disability was severely limiting my activities and forcing me to give up being the person I had known myself to be my entire life.

As a thrill seeker, I was at odds with myself. I didn't know who to be. I was pursuing the biggest thrill of my life: seeing in 3D. I didn't know who I would become when I could see in 3D. I doubted I would even recognize myself.

Hermit

I became afraid of leaving the house and going to familiar places in case I'd get overwhelmed, tired and confused.

I was much happier when I was traveling as opposed to how stuck I felt when I was going to VT thrice weekly and did no traveling. But I realized that being away from home and my routine actually made me less consistent. What I needed was for my brain to be relaxed so it could absorb the changes it was going through. My comings and goings nationally or internationally were anything but calm.

I developed into more and more of a hermit. I just couldn't stand noise or being in a place with several people speaking at once. I canceled dinners, parties and social gatherings. Music at the gym and at cafes bothered me.

Having a lot more free time due to my reduced social activities meant I spent more time at home reading books and watching movies. I watched more movies and read more books than ever in my life. Luckily, my double vision flared up only rarely when I was reading. It was my way of traveling while my brain adapted to rewiring itself to see in stereo.

Giving up myself

Becoming a hermit, I felt like I was giving up who I was. Watching Julia Roberts in the movie *Eat, Pray, Love,* reinforced my frustration. I was in the anger stage of the grieving process and my inability to be myself frustrated me immensely. Since I was periodically seeing in double, both she and actor Javier Bardem were in duplicate on the big screen. They were both such beauties that it wasn't too bad to see them with two noses, but it did distract me from the movie.

The movie was an adaptation of Elizabeth Gilbert's memoir by the same name. I was moved during the scene in the ashram where she realized that God resided in her as who she was, not by her attempt to be some super quiet pious meditator. The movie got me thinking about how much of myself I had been holding back because of binocular vision therapy. Perhaps I was trying too hard to be the dutiful patient. Staying in one place and going to the doctor religiously two to three times a week was counter to who I was: a traveler. In the movie and in the book, the protagonist got a divorce because the marriage wasn't allowing her to be who she wanted to be: child-free and a free spirit. My vision therapy sometimes left me feeling handcuffed because of the fatigue, double vision and other side effects that prevented me from traveling or being social.

In general, I felt stuck. What I was seeking was a new way of seeing the world; however, what I was experiencing was being limited. When I complained about my situation, I didn't want to sound like the complainers who didn't take responsibility for their lives. I was aware that I had gotten myself into VT. However, I had never experienced so many ups and downs with my energy levels and inability to focus for long periods of time. There were times when I just let go of my ambition and said, "Take it day by day," and then several days later, I teared up when

I saw something in double or realized I didn't have the energy to do what I wanted to do.

Serious vision therapy and the traveling lifestyle do not go together. But I had to find a way to reconcile them both in my life. I had dedicated much of the first year of VT entirely to my vision, but I hadn't let my eyes adore any new sights in the world. I saw the world through travelogues I read at the gym, when I went to the gym in the quiet hours with few other patrons. What I preferred was to be traveling rather than reading other people's stories.

Losing independence

The underlying issue concerning my frustration with my slow movement towards binocularity was that I was losing my independence, energy and spirit. More than anything, the loss of my sovereignty was killing me as I had to depend on other people to drive me places. I had been the solo traveler for years, fiercely guarding my independence.

I wondered if part of what I needed to get over mentally was that I had to give up doing things alone. The whole point of my therapy was to get my brain to accept the images from both of my eyes at the same time and fuse them and not just give me the independent images of each eye separately. What bothered me about being dependent on others was that they did things on their own time, not when I wanted to go to events or be somewhere specific. I had to wait until they could drive me. It was similar to my eyes: when I saw in double, I saw objects in two different places. My eyes were like me and the person I was waiting to drive me somewhere. We were not in the same place at the same time when I needed to go somewhere.

Re-reading "Fixing My Gaze"

To make sense of my limitations and side effects, I re-read Sue Barry's *Fixing My Gaze* and it helped me a great deal to understand what I was going through.

I read it for the first time in the summer of 2009, six months before doing VT. There were many things that I simply could not understand back then because she was describing visual changes that were foreign concepts. Barry also had sensory overload and needed a lot of quiet time. It was amazing to read about the people who had their first 3D experiences and how they were so awed. One woman stopped eating her salad after her tomato looked like it was popping out of the salad! Another stayed at home and didn't read, go to work, watch TV or read on the computer. I wondered what it would be like when this would happen to me. I had already significantly limited my life. How else would I have to restrain myself?

Like the first time I read her book, I cried a lot while re-reading the hardbound volume. It wasn't a sad book, it was that it touched me so deeply because I could understand parts of it and was struggling to "get" other sections. The neuro-scientific details were difficult intellectually and I had to read certain passages two or three times or read them aloud to better understand them.

Commenter #1

I, too, went back and read parts of her book again after about seven months of going though VT. I am beginning to see in 3D but keep double guessing myself.

Notes to the reader:

I wrote this chapter to warn potential VT patients and their friends and family what could happen with VT. I am reporting my experiences and those of other VT patients who have told me their trials and tribulations. Experiences may vary. Patients may have fewer or more side effects than I did. Some other side effects could include nausea, the inability to be in a moving vehicle and debilitating diplopia while reading. The only side effect I knew about before doing VT was double vision. You could experience other side effects I haven't listed. Don't expect the optometrist or vision therapist to warn you of what might happen to you. They might not know. My sensitivity to language is an idiosyncracy based on my interests and language abilities. Someone else doing VT may find another habitual activity become more challenging.

Approach VT knowing that your life may change significantly, not just your vision. VT is not like taking yoga or pilates three times a week. You are rewiring your brain and forcing it to do what it has resisted doing your entire life. Imagine moving the synapses in your brain to a new location to elicit different reactions. The result is that your brain may fight very hard to change or resist change, resulting in major fatigue, personality changes and other side effects. When I said this to a friend, she said I was like my own mental plumber!

Chapter Four

Explaining the Unexplainable

It is a Thursday evening around rush hour. We walk in the Berkeley BART (train) station and go through the turnstiles and descend the stairs to the platform. I put my right hand on the handrail of the staircase, carefully and slowly moving my feet step-by-step. Other commuters are practically running down the stairs without looking.

"You know, there are lots of germs on that handrail. Why are you holding the handrail?" he asks.

Restraining my anger, I say, "Didn't you hear me in the restaurant? I told you it's hard for me to walk down stairs. I don't see depth. I need to hold the handrail because otherwise I might fall. It's hard for me to see when one step ends and the other one starts."

I am embarrassed to have just admitted my disability to anyone within earshot of me in the busy train station.

I don't want to get angry with him right now in the train station in front of everybody.

He had never heard of limited depth perception until just an hour ago when I told him about it as we were sitting in a Turkish restaurant. He asked me why I came to Berkeley every Thursday. I told him about my vision therapy, the scarcity of VT doctors, and the sacrifice it was for me to have to wake up early and fight traffic to get to the train to get to Berkeley by 9 am every Thursday—a two hour journey. I also opened up about how I hadn't been working for a while because the therapy had so many side effects, which made me tired. As I sat eating my chicken sandwich and drinking my Ajran yogurt, tears came to my eyes, tears I rarely showed anybody. I had cried about this many times on my own, but I felt comfortable showing these tears to him.

"You know, my life has been on hold for several years. There are so many things that I've been wanting to do and I can't do," I said.

I told him how I'd sometimes wake up crying, just wanting to know when this would be over, when my vision would be stable. He held my hand as I talked. I told him about how I hesitated to look for work, given how sensitive I was to noise and my other limitations. I became vulnerable. He lent me an ear. He seemed to really want to understand what was going on with me. Though the owner in the restaurant knew me because I had been to this restaurant many times before, she saw me cry for the first time.

An hour later, walking down the stairs of the BART station, I feel deceived. I had just told him at the restaurant, "I can't see distance. I walk slowly down stairs because I can't see the distance from one step to the other." It seems natural to me that if I had told him I have trouble seeing distance and that I walk slowly down the stairs, that it wouldn't surprise him that my right hand would be gripping the handrail for me to sense where I am in space to protect me from falling. I always have hand sanitizer in my bag so germs are not an issue. I'd rather get the germs than fall down the stairs of a busy train station in rush hour traffic.

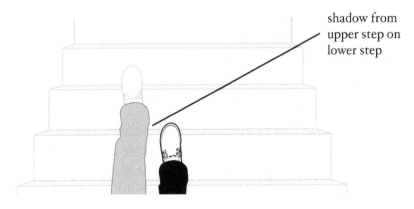

shadow from upper step on lower step

For someone who doesn't see in depth, the distance from one step to another can be hard to judge.

137

What I am seeking is to be understood, for people to listen, remember and make accommodations. The reality is that few listen, remember and change their behavior. But instead of being understood and remembered, I feel ignored, almost as though I had never said anything at all.

I have few regrets in life. One of them is not having visited Syria before the war broke out in 2011. Another major one is that I opened up to too many people in my life about my vision and vision therapy. I don't know how I would have survived withholding information about my visual changes from people around me. However, it might have been better living with pent-up emotions and impressions than dealing with the terrible outcomes I faced with the vulnerability of exposing myself.

One could very correctly argue that if I hadn't gone through so many emotional hardships on my path to improve my depth perception, I would not have written this book.

This chapter may be hard to read for those in my life whose comments and actions have hurt me. They meant no ill, but they simply didn't understand the nature of living with 2D vision or the process of VT. It is not that I didn't have people in my life who wanted to help me and be supportive; I believe they all sincerely wanted to be of assistance, but they didn't know how. Those who had gone through VT or other neurological therapies were often the ones who understood me the best. What I have written here had to be said to show how even well-meaning supporters can unknowingly hurt, offend and disrespect VT patients. Other VT patients have told me that they too have had to censor what they say about their vision because they are not understood.

My intention in this chapter is to show what it is like to discuss something others don't understand and have never heard about. The aim is to aid those with limited depth perception in knowing what to avoid and expect in communicating and for those around them to explore the emotions their 2D friends may have around the quandary of explaining the unexplainable. Those who are supporting people with limited depth perception can become aware of how to be sensitive to our situations and avoid the mistakes my well-meaning friends and family committed. Hopefully my pitfalls can help other people with binocular vision issues avoid the hurt I have felt.

The Japanese-speaking dog effect

Two Caucasian friends of mine in the U.S. both told me the same story about when they had lived in small rural Japanese towns.

When these white Americans spoke in fluent Japanese in rural Japan, many of the Japanese individuals they met looked at them and couldn't believe that these *gaijin* (foreigners) spoke Japanese. Both of my friends said to me "It was as though we were talking dogs," because of course, dogs don't talk. They bark. Seeing a white person speaking in Japanese was mind boggling. Of course, in the center of Tokyo, it was not as uncommon to see a non-Japanese person speak Japanese. But in small towns, it was exotic. In these instances, my friends said that people would respond to them in English or just not talk to them at all.

This feeling of being like an alien came back to me whenever I talked to people about what it was like for me not to see in three dimensions. I felt like the talking dog, except I wasn't speaking in Japanese. I was speaking in English or whatever language I was using to communicate. I was met with stares and questions.

"How do you survive and not fall off curbs?"

"You can't see any distance between the wall and me? We look like one image?"

"How do you drive?"

"Are you an anomaly of nature?"

"That sounds really boring and terrible. I couldn't imagine life if everything were flat."

People looked at me and they couldn't believe what I was saying. They had questions in their eyes. Their eyebrows went up. It was as though I were a talking dog. They had never met anyone like me. What I said and what I looked like didn't compute. Since my eyes looked to be cosmetically straight, explaining that I had asymmetric eyes was my first hurdle. Many did not understand that even though my eyes appeared symmetric, they weren't. The next major leap for my listeners was to understand that although I drove and did other activities requiring hand-eye coordination, I compensated for my lack of depth perception by using shadows and relative size of objects to judge distances.

Saying I could see with only one eye evoked images of Cyclops but I wasn't the one-eyed monster from Greek mythology.

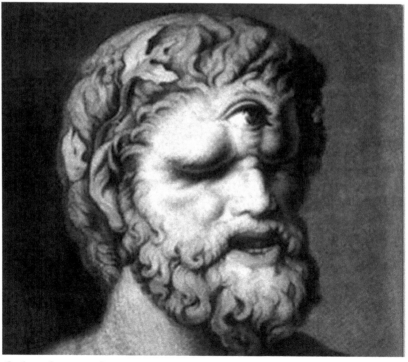

Cyclops, the one-eyed monster
Image credit: Johann Heinrich Wilhelm Tischbein, Polyphemus, 1802,
Landesmuseum Oldenburg, Germany

To explain how I wasn't Cyclops but still couldn't see with both eyes, I'd use a real life example by showing a billboard or streetlight with a building behind it.

"I don't see any distance between the billboard and that apartment building even though they are 10 feet (3 meters) apart from each other."

"Wait, you don't see any distance? How do you know the advertisement is not on the building?"

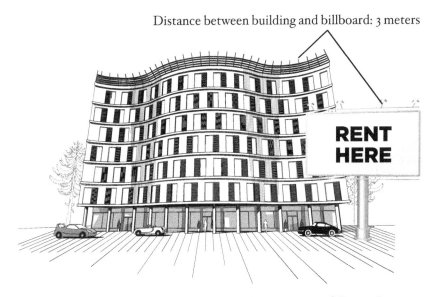

A person who can't see depth may not perceive the three meters of distance between the building and billboard. It may look like the billboard is on the building, like in this image.

"Life experience. But sometimes, I am confused because there are advertisements on buildings. I have to closely examine what I see and look for shadows or other objects between the sign and the building to see if the sign is in fact away from or on the building."

I felt like there was something wrong with my world. I had lived in this world my whole life. It's not like I was living in a still photograph. As a matter of fact, I had seen more places in the world than most of the people with normal vision who told me they thought my life was boring because I could only see in two dimensions.

My main goal in pursuing vision therapy wasn't that I thought there was something wrong with my world. I was quite happy with my world before I found out that I couldn't see like others did. I decided to do vision therapy because I wanted my life to be easier and see what other people could see. I wanted to see this other dimension. I wanted it to be easier to drive. I wanted it to be easier to park. I wanted to be able to walk down the stairs without so much difficulty. I wanted to be able to judge distances. But in the looks and stares of disbelief from others to whom I had told about my disability, I felt like there was something wrong. I felt embarrassed.

Tongue-tied polyglot

Often more difficult than VT itself was understanding what I was seeing and feeling and expressing it to others. Being a highly verbal person, it was beyond strange to experience something that I could barely understand, much less explain. I found myself staring at my fruit bowl, noticing that the orange and lime peels seemed more defined, their little circles seemed more "X," lacking the words to describe what "X" was. Like the verse in the song, *River of Dreams*, I was looking for something undefined.

My job was to help people learn other languages with ease so they could communicate with others and not feel like they had to speak like a Neanderthal or be like Tarzan beating their hands on their chest. Ironically, I was the one who felt like Tarzan. When I spoke about how wonderful it was to discover the texture of toilet paper, friends and family would laugh at me, wondering how I could seriously be excited about toilet paper.

Is my vision as cuckoo as Picasso's paintings?

A few years before I had discovered the Dalí painting, *The Hallucinogenic Toreador* (the one I described in the introduction depicting double vision), I had gone with my parents and friends to the Pablo Picasso exhibit at the De Young Museum in San Francisco. My vision seemed to come up when viewing the paintings of famous Spanish painters, even though the paintings showed disfigured faces and bodies.

Pointing to Picasso's *Three Figures Under a Tree*, my friend Anastasia said, "Is this how you see people in 2D?"

"I don't see everything in cubes like Picasso painted. But I see flat," I responded.

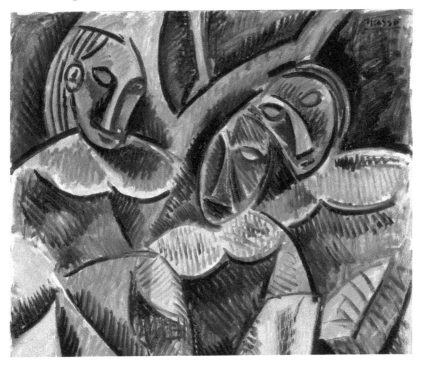

Pablo Picasso, "Three Figures under a tree"
© 2015 Estate of Pablo Picasso / Artists Rights Society (ARS), New York

Then she pointed to another image of a curvy woman. (Picasso had many wives, mistresses and muses. He painted many breasts, butts and other round body parts of various people.)

"Do you see people's curves like in this painting?" Anastasia inquired.

"No, not this flat. I do see that a woman's breasts are not as flat as in a painting."

I struggled to explain my sight since I didn't know what 3D was yet.

Later, I saw a painting of another of Picasso's many female interests, Dora Maar. He painted her nose with the nostrils separated, as though there were two noses. Her eyes were also noticeably far from each other. When I saw someone in double,

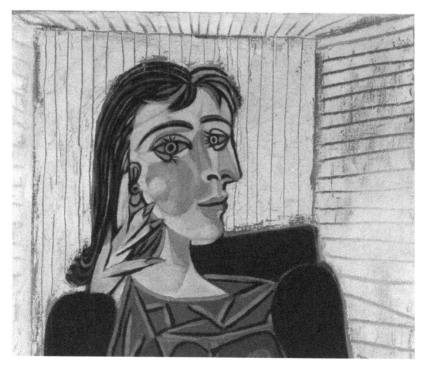

Pablo Picasso, "Portrait of Dora Maar"
© 2015 Estate of Pablo Picasso / Artists Rights Society (ARS), New York

this was sort of like how they appeared. Their features were distorted.

The inability to have a common language with most people about vision meant that I was also reticent to share my glories. When I had seen the magnificent fumes of cigarette smoke in Chinatown, I wasn't going to stop a tourist about to take a photo underneath the dragons at the Chinatown Gate and say, "Hey, can you see that cloud of lung cancer smoke across the street? Isn't that cool?" when I knew very well that tourists didn't come to one of the most visited cities in the world to admire people ingesting carcinogenic fumes. The same happened when I wanted to bask in the beauty of the small drops of water in my neighbor's sprinklers or flies in the park. Explaining what I was seeing would deplete my energy and take away the magic.

When the snowfall in Armenia had fascinated me, I asked the person I was walking with to just let me stand for a bit to admire the snow, but he wanted to keep on walking. I didn't feel comfortable explaining why I wanted to just stand in the cold and look at the snow.

I recalled my nephew when he was two-years old and he saw a fountain at a store in Big Sur and yelled, in Russian, *вода* (water)! I also wanted to exclaim, "Rain! Snow! Toilet paper! Flies!" each time I saw some "banal" element of life spring out towards me in all of its glory. But I would have felt like a total fool because I wasn't a two-year-old who had seen a fountain for the first time.

Invisible crutches = lack of understanding

I rarely had still points of reference like the Dalí and Picasso paintings to use to explain my situation and I had to allude to a moving picture.

The rift between me and those around me was crossed only by those who also had an unexplainable issue.

In 1992, I saw the movie *Damage* with Jeremy Irons and Juliette Binoche; the story was about a British Parliament member having an affair with his son's girlfriend. The plot aside, what I recalled from the movie was when Binoche told Irons that they could both understand each other because they were both "damaged."

This scene from the movie came to me when I was telling a friend why I thought he didn't comprehend my feeling hurt when friends and family didn't understand how important VT was to me. Maybe only someone who, like me, had sacrificed everything for something (i.e. VT) and had not yet reached their goal, could appreciate my frustration. Stereoptic vision was the only thing in my life that I had dreamed of, worked harder than anything else to achieve, and had not yet attained after five arduous years of exercises, a depleting bank account, and lost friendships. One didn't need to be an adult strabismic to empathize. Any other hard working overachiever who had not reached their goals could feel my pain.

Some friends and family inquired as to why I hadn't just dropped the whole "VT thing" if it was causing me so many debilitating side effects. I wasn't a quitter, nor did I ever intend to become one. Letting go of my dream was not a possibility; I knew I needed to keep at it. Plus, my ophthalmologist told me that because of my intermittent double vision, if I gave up VT, I'd have to wear a visible patch on one eye (like a pirate's patch) to make my brain go back to using just one eye at a time. I was afraid I'd lose the gains in acuity and my beloved flies and dust if I turned back. I was in limbo.

This reader's comment to this entry resonated well with me.

Commenter #3:

I, too, have spent years in vision therapy, watched two of my children succeed and have yet to see any real progress. When my husband asks me what I want in life, I can't even tell him that what I really want is stereovision. (I've said it before.) He tells me I am beautiful despite my eye turn, but I just want my eyes to be straight and see one image. I'm glad you continue to blog.

Those who could best understand what I was going through, besides those that I knew who had gone through vision therapy, were those who had done other intensive therapy. One friend was a recovering alcoholic and was going to Alcoholics Anonymous and Codependents Anonymous meetings. Her struggles with not drinking were a daily phenomenon. She couldn't tell people at work why she was having trouble concentrating. Another friend was doing cancer therapy and despite his repeated explanations to his coworkers about why he needed help with certain physical tasks, his coworkers still didn't "get it" and would constantly ask him to do things he had told them he couldn't do.

If I had been walking around with crutches it would have been obvious that I wasn't as mobile or agile as most people. But because my therapy was inside my head and could not be seen (ironic, eh?), few could appreciate and recall that I was in fact not as energetic or available as before. It was a pain to have to keep reminding people why I couldn't do things. I wished they would just cut me some slack or leave me alone.

My inner crutches were evident only to me, my doctor and others who have had to somehow "re-wire" themselves.

My family member asked me twice to drive her to sweltering Sacramento to see her best friend after I had previously denied her ridiculous request to drive for two hours in the heat. Her friend insisted that she ask me to drive her. I criticized this family member for not remembering that I had always hated driving and I was not in a position to drive much because of my vision and fatigue. She refused to think about my position and how much I had been going through to improve my sight. She and perhaps many others to whom I had spoken to about my vision, simply could not fathom what it was like to have to constantly negotiate with one's vision.

This constant double-checking and negotiating reality vs. perception was *extremely* tiring and nerve-racking.

I know I am searching for something,
Something so undefined
That it can only be seen
By the eyes of the blind

Advice = horse manure

The impact of speaking to people who had never heard of 2D vision was I got unsolicited and useless advice.

When I was about nine or ten years old, I had a friend, LeAnne, from Australia and we lived in the same condominium complex in San Jose. LeAnne loved horseback riding and wanted to have her own horse. Her parents sometimes took her for horseback riding lessons. While reading the newspaper's classified section, I saw advertisements for free horse manure. Not knowing the meaning of the word 'manure,' I thought, "Oh, wow, somebody's giving away a free horse." I clipped out the advertisement and called LeAnne.

"LeAnne, I have great news for you. I found you a free horse," I said, happy to be helping her.

She was very excited because she obviously wanted to have a horse. Then I read her the advertisement: "Free horse manure. Call this number XXX-XXXX."

"That's not a free horse. That's free horse *manure*," she said, annoyed.

Embarrassed because I didn't know what the word "manure" meant, I realized from the tone of her voice that I had made a mistake, but I didn't know what it was. I just said, "Oh, I'm sorry," and I changed the subject. Later, when I learned that I had offered her horse feces instead of a real horse, I was embarrassed.

That was what it was like for me when people with the best of intentions gave me advice about my vision, but they didn't know what they were talking about, just like I didn't know what the word "manure" meant.

I was in the anger stage of the five stages of grief, and I would get deeply angry with useless, but well-meant, advice. My friend's boyfriend told me, "Oh, you know, you should speak to my laser eye surgeon. He did great laser eye surgery on me." I explained to him that my issue could not be solved with laser surgery. Mine was not just a muscular issue, but also a neurological issue that could not be changed with a couple lasers in a few minutes. Even after I said, "Many optometrists do not deal with this issue. There are only a very few specialized optometrists around the world who deal with binocular vision issues," I would get passed off to somebody's casual acquaintance who was an optometrist or ophthalmologist. Others would ask why I traveled so far to see a doctor when, according to them, there had to be plenty of great eye doctors at Stanford Medical Center, 25 minutes from my house. No matter how many times I explained that Stanford did not have an optometry school specializing in this field, the same good-willed "advisors" would come back repeatedly with the same futile advice.

One person, trying to understand what I meant by double vision, 2D vision, vibrating walls and my visual progress, told me I should take photos of what I see so she could understand. I had to remind her, a photographer, that photos were only 2D and that I couldn't take a photo to show how my brain interpreted depth. My photo wouldn't show people with two nosess and three eyes or my vibrating bathroom floor. The photos, unless digitally modified, would only show what the camera "saw" at a specific moment in time, not what my brain interpreted. When I had to point out the blatantly obvious, my frustration mounted even more and I just wanted to stop talking about my condition.

The worst advice I got was when people, upon hearing about my eye issue, heard the words "eye" and "vision issue" and automatically thought of carrots and told me I should eat more carrots because the Vitamin A in carrots helps the eyes. I could have eaten a field of carrots and the only thing that would have changed about me was that I would have looked like a big orange monster! Carrots were not an easy fix for a VT patient learning to move their eyes in harmony and doing exercises to stretch their eye muscles so their eyes would be aligned. Carrots would not wake up dormant binocular brain cells. If carrots had a binocular power, I would have bought a carrot farm a long time ago and sold binocular carrot supplements to the 3% of the population with amblyopia and strabismus and made my bank account happy. This kind of advice trivialized my condition.

Sometimes I wouldn't show that I was upset because I knew that what the people were saying was meant to help me. What I learned was that just trying to help when someone didn't know what they're talking about could make the situation even worse.

My "advisors" thought they were helping me get my free horse, but I felt overloaded with a growing mound of benevolently-donated horse excrement. To tell my well-wishers that they were giving me horse dung instead of my beloved equestrian dream would have been crushing for them. I would have had to explain, for the umpteenth time, that their advice was not at all helpful and just like horse ≠ horse manure, limited depth perception ≠ glaucoma, cataracts, macular degeneration or whatever ocular issue their neighbor had.

When I did tell some people that their "advice" was not helping me, they promptly got defensive and said I wasn't being grateful.

This communication issue is a fundamental problem that happens with people who have hidden disabilities. When we speak to people who don't understand what we're talking about, they look within the context of their world and the circle of the people they know for somebody who has something similar. They try to equate us with that person. They try to put us in a box. But when the hidden disability doesn't fit into any of the boxes that the person has in mind, they don't know what to do with the information. It's like when you're cleaning out your closet and you want to put everything in the right drawer, but there's just that one item that doesn't fit. It's not a sock, it's not a shirt, it's not a scarf, it's not a shoe, it's something else and you have no place for it.

It wasn't one person's single advice; it was the compilation of irrelevant information day after day, month after month. All of this unwanted and useless advice just grew into a huge pile of horse manure and stunk to the high heavens. The advice was just fertilizing my ever-growing frustration! The "advisers" were trying to fix something they couldn't fix, when all I needed was for them to listen, be supportive and remember my limitations.

I had mental flashes of the scene in the movie *White Nights*, when Mikhail Barishnikov, a Soviet ballet dancer who had defected to the US, was so frustrated with being back in the former USSR and having to whisper and hide what he was feeling. Speaking to his former girlfriend (played by Helen Mirren) on the stage of the Bolshoi Theatre in Leningrad, he shouts, "I won't whisper what I feel. I want to scream. I can't lie anymore." He then does an improvised dance on the stage to the renegade music of Vladimir Vissotsky. I just wanted to tell people how I felt without having to hide or sometimes even lie about what was really going on.

I knew the advice came from ignorance and not out of ill will. I learned how annoying it could be to hear unsolicited and uninformed medical advice from a well-meaning person. Long before doing VT, I had made the same mistake.

Mark, a diabetic friend, and I were on our way to a wedding. Mark asked me to drive him to a soda machine because his glucose levels were low. I told him he should have monitored his blood sugar level before I picked him up from the airport and bought a soda there. It turned out that what I knew about diabetes from the diabetics I knew didn't pertain to Mark's situation and need for immediate sugar. My lecturing caused a disagreement between us and tension the next day when we attended the wedding. Later on Mark sent me a video made by a diabetic man telling people to stop giving him advice on his diabetes if they didn't know what they were talking about. When I saw the video, I understood that my preconceptions about diabetes did not apply to everyone with the disease. Giving unsolicited medical advice when not trained is not only dangerous but extremely insulting to the person who has to hear it. What Mark needed from me was my patience and support for his diabetes, not my advice.

A few years after the soda incident, when friends, acquaintances and family barraged me with useless suggestions about my vision problem, I emailed Mark and apologized again, telling him that I now knew how he felt when I had bothered him about his soda. I was now in his shoes, lacking the empathy of others.

By the time I discovered the section on how to deflect unwanted advice in the book *Living Well with a Hidden Disability,* it was already too late. I had been burned and bruised by horse manure and I distanced myself from people who had either hurt or annoyed me with their misguided advice or comments. Sometimes I even completely ended friendships. (A description of *Living Well With a Hidden Disability* is in the Resources section at the end of this book.)

Wonders of VT remind me of a *Sex in the City* episode

Despite the lack of a common language between most of my friends and me, my struggles with fatigue and headaches were not completely ignored.

My challenges reminded me of the "A Woman's Right to Shoes" episode in HBO's popular series, *Sex and the City,* in which Carrie Bradshaw (Sarah Jessica Parker) lamented that as a single woman without children, she never got any gifts or cards to celebrate moments in her life, unlike her married friends with kids who received bridal shower, wedding and baby shower presents.

"You don't get a Hallmark card that says, 'Congratulations for not marrying the wrong man'," Carrie said, exasperated.

There were also no parties, Hallmark cards, or generally recognized moments of congratulations for when VT patients stared at granules of salt on the white part of a boiled egg because suddenly they could perceive small white specs of salt on a white surface—an effort requiring a level of visual acuity they previously didn't have. There were no "let's admire flying dust particles in the sunlight" summer barbecues. There was no Meetup group for vision therapy patients to go on hikes and stare at trees and rock back and forth underneath them to revel in the distance between the branches. (I did try to organize a meeting for adult strabismic people in the Bay Area but it didn't work out.)

The day after I wrote this blog post about the *Sex and the City* episode, Luis and a group of friends organized a surprise party to show their support for what I was going through in VT. It turned out that my difficulties were not completely unappreciated. I was deeply moved and wrote this poem as a thank you:

Bespectacled or with naked divergent eyes

Blinded she was to Luis's surprise

Being a medical mystery

Brought her much misery

Ten plus medical professionals with many degrees

Couldn't make her smile like karaoke and Javier's brie cheese

For what are friends for

if not to make one's spirit soar?

It's good to know that compassion

is not going out of fashion

My brain and eyes are rewiring

and the love of friends and family is inspiring

In stereo I will see

With or without a Harvard PhD's guarantee*

*I had gone to see a Harvard Medical School PhD in neuro-ophthalmology the previous year at UCSF who told me (diplomatically) that I was a lost cause.

Further intensifying my frustration was that, despite friends' efforts to cheer me up with a party, I still felt deep isolation because when I spoke to them about my situation, I felt they couldn't grasp what I was experiencing. From the outside, it looked like I should not have felt so lonely and misunderstood, but I did. It was hard to voice my disappointment with some friends and family because, in their minds, they were doing what they could do to raise my spirits and I was grateful for their efforts. However, there was still a powerful disconnect between what I was struggling with and how little they understood and remembered.

Splitting myself into two

The song *Debo partirme en dos* (I have to split myself into two) by the Cuban singer-songwriter Silvio Rodríguez came to mind when I realized that I may have a double life: one with VT and one where I pretended my vision was not an issue. I got so tired of explaining myself that I figured that hiding the truth might be a better option than being open and honest.

This song is about a musician in Cuba whose concert might be cancelled and who is often misunderstood. I am assuming Rodríguez is making reference to the Communist government of Cuba censuring his work. Despite this song not being health-related, it resonated with me because I also felt that I was better off censoring myself and having a double life. Given that many in VT experience double vision, which they must learn to fuse into a singular binocular image, this song touched more than one chord with me.

Below are the original lyrics in Spanish, the English translation and my comments.

Spanish	English translation	Comments
No se crean que es majadería.	*Do not think that is nonsense.*	Don't think my vision issues are nonsense
Que nadie se levante aunque me ría.	*Nobody is getting up even though they are making fun of me*	I have been explaining my disability to the incredulous for years
Hace rato que vengo lidiando con gente que dice que yo canto cosas indecentes.	*It's been a while that I've been arguing/ fighting with people who say that I sing indecent things.*	But they don't understand the fantastical world I describe.
Debo partirme en dos	*I have to split myself into two*	I have to split myself into two: the one who struggles in VT and the one who can't talk about it
Unos dicen que aquí,	*Some say here*	One eye goes here, another eye goes there
otros dicen que allá	*others say there*	
y sólo quiero decir,	*and I just want to say*	
sólo quiero cantar	*I just want to sing*	I just want to do this therapy and see in 3D
y no importa la suerte	*it doesn't matter*	
que pueda correr una canción.	*how successful this song will be*	
...	*...*	
y no importa que luego	*and never mind that*	Just respect that I am where I am, even if I fail
me suspendan la función	*later my concert will be cancelled*	

No voy a repetir ese estrebrillo	*I will not repeat that chorus*	I am sick and tired of explaining myself and being misinterpreted.
...	...	...
y estoy temiendo ahora no ser interpretado:	*I fear now that I will be misinterpreted*	
casi siempre sucede que se piensa algo malo	*Almost always, people think something wrong.*	
Debo partirme en dos.	*I have to split myself in two*	I have to split myself in two

Silencing myself, not finding empathy

I understood that sometimes it was better to just be quiet, but it felt fundamentally unfair. I was probably in the depression stage of grief.

A fellow amblyope told me, when I lamented the lack of understanding around me, "It's just not in their reality."

Other people in my life had issues which I had listened to and understood, even if their situations were not part of my reality, but mine was completely out of their grasp. For example, I felt for many years like I was "Dial-a-Shrink." When people had an issue, they called me to get help because I was a good listener. A few days after meeting me, one man who had recently lost his girlfriend in a car accident, told me about his loss. I was one of the few people in our area who knew about what had happened. A dear friend who lived in a predominantly Muslim country came out to me that he was gay and I had to keep that secret, but at the same time I became his coming-out counselor. I wasn't a man, I wasn't gay, I hadn't grown up in a predominantly Muslim country, but I could help him because I knew—from my other homosexual friends—what it was like to come out. Other people confided in me about their issues, whether they were dealing with insomnia, an addiction problem, divorce, bankruptcy or losing their home. One friend's son was arrested. I didn't have any children and I definitely didn't have any children who had been arrested. I knew what these subjects were just from being a person in society, from reading, from having other people in my life who had similar issues. I could lend a helpful ear and give relevant advice, if that's what friends requested, based on my experience and what I knew.

When it came time for me to need a helping ear, somebody who would listen carefully and remember the details about what I had said, I found that there were very few people I could count on to be the person that I had been for them when they needed help. I felt cheated. I had been a very private person and people had told me, "You know, you need to share more. You need to be more effusive." I somehow envied people who were more extroverted, who could just freely talk about what was going on in their lives. Incidentally, it was precisely those who wanted me to be more effusive who were the worst listeners, forgetting what I had told them about limited depth perception. I realized I was a natural empath, but though my listening brought catharsis to others, the majority of those around me were anything but empathetic.

I had met many strangers on buses, planes, and other places who confided deep secrets about what was going on with them. I thought, very naively so, that if I were just like them, if I just freely shared what was happening with me, that other people would listen to me like I had been listening to them and I'd feel a catharsis.

I could not have been more wrong. It was precisely my unconscious expectation that made my life so difficult. As I needed to talk about what was happening with my vision, I opened up and I told people—not random people at the supermarket, but people in my life—friends, colleagues, acquaintances. Sometimes people would change the subject quickly, look at something else, or their gaze would move or they would roll their eyes. I heard later on from some that they could not understand what was happening with me. My explanations of why I could suddenly see dust that I couldn't see before didn't make any sense to them because they had seen dust their entire lives.

Deep down, I felt that I had really gotten the short end of the stick. All these years I had counseled people on their issues, listened until 2:00 or 3:00 in the morning as they talked about what was happening with them, even when I had to get up early the next morning. I would then spend the following day very tired because I had been up so late listening and talking. But now, when it was my time to need help, to make sense of the world that was changing before me, I could count on only a few people who would really be there for me, whom I could call and talk to in the middle of the night if I needed to. I felt like I might be overburdening the few people who did have a sympathetic ear. That extreme loneliness made the whole situation worse.

Being more open about what was happening with me turned out to be a colossal mistake, because in being more open, I became incredibly and painfully vulnerable. Not being met by a sympathetic ear, somebody who could empathize with what I was going through, I felt that what I had to contribute about what was happening in my life wasn't necessarily as important as what other people had going on. I felt very self-conscious about sharing. It seemed silly to talk about dust, flies, rain, snow and mold. It was much easier to write in my blog and to a few VT email pen pals. In this desire to be more open, I actually had to become more closed. It was a coping mechanism.

Reading about other people with hidden disabilities in the book *Living Well With a Hidden Disability*, I realized I actually wasn't the only person going through this. Anytime somebody has symptoms or a situation that doesn't fall into the norm or what people have heard about on *Dr. Oz* or *Oprah* or in their high school biology class, they can't understand it. Since they can't understand it, they usually don't remember what's been said. This, unfortunately, is something that I have yet to resolve. I am still quite guarded about what I say because I have to filter my audience and realize to whom it is worth disclosing my reality.

Help from readers

The VT blogging was a true lifeline to keep me from feeling even more lonely.

In the blog, I asked readers who had amblyopia for advice on how to deal with unwanted questions. One reader, Commenter #11, said:

> *No good at deflecting here. Unfortunately, it comes up a lot, since I don't highway drive, and rely on my husband a lot. Now that my eyes are cosmetically corrected, it's even harder to explain...*

Out of utter frustration after an argument with my mother about why I was celebrating my birthday alone, in silence, instead of in a loud festive atmosphere, I asked readers to give me their advice on how to deal with people who refuse to accept our disability and limitations. This question became one of the most interactive threads in the blog and helped me see that I was far from alone in my irritation.

> *Commenter #8 says:*
>
> *I never got the operation so I definitely don't look "normal." Even in my case my friends and family don't seem to really*

accept that my eyes have had a dramatic effect on the way I see the world and on the way the world sees me. During my VT work last year I found myself often engaging friends on the subject of how the world looks to me. Most really weren't that interested. Sometimes they were weirded out but mostly they just didn't find it too interesting.

In retrospect, I think I understand. One friend of mine is in Alcoholics Anonymous. When she first joined it colored her entire world view, she worked it into every conversation, every bad thing that happened in our town was due, in her view, to a "drunk." This was certainly the way she saw the world and she is a dear friend but it stopped being a two-way conversation. She was no longer conversing with me. I'm going to try to keep that example in my mind when I am tempted to bring up my eyes more than, say, once… unless someone asks.

This is really tough, and it's lonely, but it's important to cut other people a lot of slack. (Really, not just about our eyes. More slack is needed in our world.) They have their own stuff that they can't talk about. Oh, the stuff people live with! And we can maybe identify with them a little more because we have our eyes.

As far as the noisy environment issue, well, I'm with you all the way. I'm certainly not tolerant of it now. It seems related to multitasking and I can't do that at all anymore and it drives me crazy to have two people talking at me. Yuck.

Commenter #13 says:

There's a positive part in me that doesn't accept the simple fact that I've got a good eye there and don't use it.

Will this feeling be enough to front up to my closest relatives when therapy takes so long and it's so terribly expensive?

I've told my mother I'm going back to where I was 30 years ago before the operation, turning strabismic again. She was surprised, and worried because, you know, in Italy we care so much for appearances. When I tell her that even after the operation my brain never learned how to use my left eye, she simply switches off.

I tell that to my father and my older sister, they're both doctors but they haven't read Sue Barry's book. So it's hard for them to imagine what it's like to be monocular, as it's just as hard for me to imagine what it's like to see depth.

Commenter #11:

I, obviously, am not who you were talking to here—but I feel like I want to run through the screen and hug you. I HATE that people don't understand monocular vision, and assume that the operation fixed it. Mine's strictly cosmetic, as well.

I don't do very well with that. I had my operation, I look normal—but I don't see in 3D. The eyes just don't work together. So driving, is a pain. As a rule, I don't drive the highway.

Merging and all, is a nightmare. I usually don't bring it up with friends, unless pressed, because no one seems to understand. Which, I can't say that I blame them. I can't imagine what looking at things with both eyes must look like...

I don't think my family gets it. My husband does, to a point. I usually just don't bother trying to explain if the people don't get it. It's frustrating, but there isn't any sense in trying further, and making myself more frustrated. :(

AND, why is it so hard to believe VT would affect other senses? The senses affect each other. You take one away, the others grow stronger. It's an easy assumption that other issues with senses, could mess with the other four.

Commenter #6 says:

Great post, thanks. My eyes usually appear straight as a result of VT. The few people who have commented have said that it makes me look "intense," "different," or even "angry!"

Only a few people have taken a sincere interest in my VT; one is an artist and the other a neuroscientist!

I also have noise sensitivity and often wear ear plugs at the dinner table. The sound of a fork hitting a plate hard just about kills me.

When I tell people I don't drive they don't believe me and never remember. I think they think I mean I try not to drive, like in an eco-friendly way. Some people, not to be outdone, claim they also don't drive—by which they mean they only drive to work, etc. I literally have not driven a car even once since the early/mid 90's! Yet people STILL think I drive.

To be honest I have basically given up on that and I actually kind of fear that if I do achieve real 3D it will seem profound to me but I will not be able to convey my feelings to friends/family, I think that will be difficult.

Commenter #13

I'm convinced about two things now:

1. Empathy really happens when you have had direct experience of someone else's feelings. It's hard to imagine what it feels like to have kidney stones, or to give birth, unless you've gone through it.

2. We lack a powerful metaphor for describing something that cannot even be drawn because it happens in binocular minds. I've started telling people: if you've never walked, you would die to walk. I think that's pretty tangible.

I responded:

I agree with you on #2. Dr. Sacks said in his first article about "Stereo Sue" that explaining 3D to a stereo-blind person is like explaining color to a blind person. You just can't.

I'm a natural empath. And if someone tells me X is difficult for them or makes them dizzy or whatever, I feel empathy for their situation. So I expect the same in my situation and this expectation is what is killing me.

Commenter #13:

I've asked the optometrist about how he explains to parents what their children with double vision see. He said he puts a prism in front of one parent's eye to cause double vision, and sometimes they cry!

I responded:

Great idea! And I'll scream in people's ears while drumming to make them aware of how noises drive me crazy and how their loud voices are irritating!

Seriously, using a prism to show someone what double vision is seems like an excellent idea. I am glad the parents cry. It makes them aware of how hard it is for their kids.

Commenter #6 says:

Regarding the prism idea, I have had people try on my prism glasses and look completely shocked—my glasses make them see double. They can't take them off fast enough. With a few people I could tell this was what finally made them accept that there was really something different about me!

I responded:

I put my prism glasses on my mom and she wanted them off in seconds! My sister's kids think it's fun to see in double through the glasses.

Commenter #5 says:

I am having my first Visual Therapy session tomorrow. I am very excited and worried about it.

I have had strabismus since I remember. I had three surgeries and my eyes are straight now most of the time. However, sometimes if I look quickly at something or at a strange angle then one of my eyes, usually the left one, wanders away.

My eyes are straight but I always felt that there is something wrong in the way I see the world. I felt a big gap between people and the way they live. I always wanted to be like one of them: easygoing, relaxed but I always had a strange feeling that I am at a lack of something.

After reading Sue Barry's book I finally found the answer.

I found what I am missing and why sometimes I act so different to others.

I tried to find a visual therapy specialist in London for the last three years but I couldn't find any. So many times I gave up and thought it is only in my head. My mother and my sister were telling me I am cured and there is nothing wrong. Telling me my eyes are straight and that is what matters.

I was very shy and neurotic before. My gaze was always focused but it was tiring me and I could not enjoy life. Then I learned to relax my gaze and body but my thoughts began to wander away as well as my eyes. I started to lose attention to people around me, to my work, to all of my previous world. And all I wanted to do was run away somewhere quiet and natural and live on a small farm or a village and enjoy small things. Life became very boring.

Sometimes I wonder if the way I see and the way I think are connected. I feel two persons in me. One is shy and neurotic and very closed minded and another is brave and maybe eager to explore the world but at the same time, he is so eliminated from real life and people around. I don't know who I am.

Maybe it is the two hemispheres of my brain trying to work together?

On my birthday and Christmas Day I asked God to help me. Then shortly after I found a link to a visual behavior optometrist with over 20 years of experience in London. I spoke to her and got very excited. I am seeing her tomorrow.

El Buenrostro (Mr. Goodface)

San Diego, California and Tijuana, Mexico April-May 2013

The US Consulate driver from Tijuana, Mexico picks me up from the San Diego Airport and we drive in silence across the busiest border crossing in the world. In Tijuana, I look at the billboards and notice one for a plastic surgeon called Dr. Buenrostro (Dr. Goodface). I can't believe the plastic surgeon was born with such a fitting surname.

The city is full of large pharmacies on the street, like fruit and vegetable stands with a roof but no doors. They look like permanent stands but they have moveable tin doors the shopkeepers use to close the business at night. Clinics and medical laboratories are working even at 9 pm on Sunday nights to handle all of the medical tourists from the US and local clients. You cannot go too far without finding a clinic that would make your nose smaller, enlarge or reduce breasts, take out unwanted fat, or perform other surgeries.

While eating sushi at an outside table in a mini mall, I see a large billboard for Colombian "fajas," post-surgical bodysuits/girdles for those recovering from liposuction and other surgeries who don't want to look flabby. Some of the bodysuits also have butt lifters to make one's rear end look extra curvy and noticeable—still a mystery to me in flatland.

After not being able to travel much because of my language confusion problems, I was very excited to go to Mexico to give educational presentations to Mexican students, teachers and college professors about learning English using music, TV, radio, movies and other media. Since I was going to have to speak to the Mexican media in live interviews and give several presentations a day in Spanish, I didn't want to overtax my brain by being social. I resigned myself to stay in my hotel room each night watching Mexican TV, getting ahead with advanced episodes of the Mexican soap opera I was following (the TV in Mexico was about a month ahead of the episodes shown in the US), quietly reading or relaxing.

On May 1st, after a live morning radio interview, I went by foot to a restaurant to eat ceviche. The city was almost deserted for the International Labor Day holiday. For much of the day, I walked alone along the mostly deserted streets and downtown area, appreciating the silence. I returned to my hotel to get ready for my trip the next day to Mexicali, another border city further east and famous for its Mexican-Chinese cuisine. I opened my email and received an invitation from a close friend, Luis, sent to our group of friends and acquaintances, inviting us to a free 3D screening of the NASA movie about Mars.

I replied to all saying that I couldn't see in 3D and wouldn't be able to appreciate the film and asked to be removed from the email thread. I was annoyed that I, again, had to remind my friends what I had said so many times. I felt like a little toddler kicking, screaming and yelling, "I want an ice cream" at a party, to get people's attention and to have them remember my situation.

About an hour later, I stood in the shower and instead of revering the small drops of moisture ascending in the mist, I felt salty tears run down my face and into my mouth.

I was boiling with anger. Luis knew full well that I couldn't see in 3D. He was actually the one who had organized my surprise party a year and a half prior to cheer me up as I was struggling so much with my vision and side effects. He had heard my descriptions of the therapy, double vision and confusion. Getting his email was a huge slap in the face. It felt like that rock salt I loved in Brazilian *churrascos* (BBQ), but this time, the rock salt was on my deep and open wounds, not on sumptuous meat.

How hard could it be to understand? He knew I couldn't see in 3D and had been suffering because of VT and the inability to fuse. How could he be so thoughtless as to invite me to a 3D movie? I know he didn't invite me deliberately to hurt me, but it showed a major lack of respect and appreciation for what I had been going through for almost three and a half years.

Finally my side effects had been getting more manageable and I was traveling and I felt great. And then boom, someone delivered a reminder of something that I couldn't do and it stung for days, weeks and months later. The tears didn't stop coming out of my already tired eyes, looking bright green with red in the white part of the eye. I had to face the reality that dealing with a hidden disability was socially challenging.

A few days after receiving the email, the consulate driver arrived in Mexicali in a bullet-proof van with super heavy doors that were hard to open and close. I was afraid I'd cut off my leg if the door slammed on me before I was completely in or out of the van. Driving from Mexicali to Tijuana, we crossed into the US to use safer roads. (The Mexican road between Mexicali and Tijuana was dangerous as drug mafias did carjackings and kidnappings on the road.) We passed harsh terrain of cactii and rocks with small water canisters left by volunteers to hydrate those people crossing illegally from Mexico into the US. Trying to keep my mind off of the 3D movie invitation, I chatted the whole time with the driver. I knew very well how lucky I was to be in an air-conditioned and bullet-proof vehicle and not crossing the border in the heat without potable water sources nearby or any signs of civilization. My logical mind told me Luis didn't intend to hurt me, but my emotions were strong and I was crying rivers inside. I wanted my heart to be as strong as the bullet-proof doors of the van so I wouldn't get hurt so easily.

The sun was setting along the Pacific Ocean as we traversed through busy Friday evening traffic in downtown San Diego to return to Mexico. Upon crossing the border, I was again met by the friendly-looking face of Dr. Carlos Buenrostro on a tall billboard, inviting patients to slim their waist, change their face or do other procedures to look better.

Someone at the consulate told me that Mr. Buenrostro had not been born with the surname "Goodface." The doctor also had to alter something about himself: his identity.

Judging from the medical tourism traffic in Tijuana, I knew many came there to change their looks. But appearances were deceiving. We can transform ourselves aesthetically to follow societal norms, but that doesn't mean we metamorphose from inside and become just like everyone else, or in my case, see just like everyone else. Would patients reducing their nose size emerge from the doctor's office accepting of him or herself, no matter the results of the surgery? Would post-rhinoplasty patients be accepting of others who chose to leave their large noses intact?

It was ironic that I was surrounded by plastic surgery clinics catering to people who want to look "normal" or "better" and inside, I was at pains with how my "looking normal" made it so easy for close friends and family to forget part of who I was.

The following comment was immensely soothing as I knew that those with 2D vision could feel how painful it was for me to receive such an inappropriate 3D movie invitation.

Commenter #12:

Hello lovely,

I'm still pretty new to the strabismic changes in my life (it's been just three years—although it feels like it's been an eternity) and one thing that I keep learning over and over is that our respective journeys are different from one another. Your entry has revealed another false assumption on my part... I really enjoy going to 3D movies... because it's the only time, so far, that I can see in 3D. I thought it was the same for all of us because the depth is created by other methods... glasses, etc... and not dependent solely on our own eyes to create the sense of depth. It's not real, but it looks real, and it feels real.

You have tried to see a movie in 3D before, right?

Is it not the same for you?

I realize now that I can make another (unexpected) point here... and I hope that you will recognize that I don't mock your pain, I acknowledge it... and OH HOW I understand it! But if someone WITH strabismus, and a clear understanding of your pain and your experience and your trial (because I walk a similar path) can still make an assumption that can cause such remorse, how much easier is it for someone who has no idea to do the same?

I too have felt the same pain, cried the same hot tears that burn my face in anguish when someone has said or done something that seemed absolutely insensitive and thoughtless. I better understand their ignorance as I realize that I too, even from a perspective of knowing personally this point of view, can make an assumption that turns out to be so far from the truth.

Through this experience, I am compelled toward two things.

First, I want to apologize... profusely... and with great depth of sincerity, for my own ignorance and insensitivity toward you. I am so very sorry, sweetheart. I assure you, it was unintentional.

Secondly, my heart is softened toward those who have, in their own ignorance, said or done something that has hurt me. And this is good, because forgiveness always brings peace. But now, I understand THEIR perspective a bit better for having had this experience.

THANK YOU for sharing your thoughts.

They have widened my perspective in unexpected and wonderful ways.

Thank you.

Note: I did try watching 3D movies with 3D glasses and I didn't see the 3D effects. I just spent extra money at the cinema to wear an extra pair of glasses and I saw nothing different than when I closed one eye and saw the film in 2D.

It is not that I always wanted to be seen as the person with _____ disability, just like artists/singers/athletes from minority groups don't want to always be seen as the "Hispanic singer" or "African American athlete," but just as a "singer" or "athlete." I often got irritated being referred to as "so and so's friend who speaks lots of languages" as though I had no other identifying attributes.

I just wanted my friends and family to think before inviting me to events or asking me to do things that required depth perception. It would have been better to preface requests or invitations by showing that they understood that the activity may not be appropriate for me but they still wanted to include me and then ask if I'd be interested or available.

A color-blind colleague told me that even though he can see in 3D, he can't see 3D movies because he doesn't see red and green and 3D movie glasses have red and green lenses. He told me he also felt embarrassed when his friends wanted to go to 3D movies.

Excuses: But You Look So Normal

As witnessed in the 3D movie episode, my "looking normal" deafened people to what I had told them about my eyes and highlighted the ways in which my understanding of respect for others was not shared.

If I had a guest coming over and I remembered that they had a certain food allergy or something that they couldn't eat, I didn't prepare food with that ingredient. It was my way of showing respect. Just like if you were to have a practicing Muslim or Jew come to your house, most likely you're not going to feed them pork chops because pork is against their religion. My unconscious assumption was that if I just told people, "Listen, I have trouble driving at night. I can't be in loud places. These are my limitations," people would remember that just as I recalled people's food allergies.

I was completely wrong.

"Remember, it's hard for me to drive at night and the reason is because in the absence of light, I have no cues for distance. I don't see the edge of a car so well when all I see are headlights. It's hard for me to judge how close or how far away a car is. If it's raining at night, forget it, because the lights move around in my visual field and I can't see," I'd repeatedly explain.

My explanations notwithstanding, I would get the same invitations to go places requiring me to drive at night. Since my vision issues fluctuated, sometimes I could drive at night or even go out dancing (for a limited period of time). I didn't announce my abilities on a daily basis like the security alerts at the airport. So my friends weren't sure of when I was able to drive or go out, causing them to sometimes overestimate my abilities. As a result, I got annoyed thinking they didn't remember. (See the Chapter Six Advice section for tips on including VT patients in social activities.)

One of my friends, a nurse practitioner, confided in me.

"The reason we often say things to you that get on your nerves or invite you to things that you can't do is that we forget that you have this disability because it's hidden."

"You're so active. You're quite accomplished. You write books. You're making a movie. It's hard for people to remember that you have to make accommodations in your daily life," she said.

"But I told people under which duress I operate and how many sacrifices I have to make in order to do things."

"Because you look normal, we don't remember."

I think what she meant by "normal" is that my eyes look symmetric and that if I hadn't told them that I had a disability, they wouldn't have known it.

I learned that other people with hidden disabilities had the same type of frustration. Because their disability was not apparent on their body, even their spouses and other family members forgot and didn't make special accommodations for them.

Indeed, it was hard for people to remember what their eyes couldn't corroborate. The bottom line was, I didn't want to have to keep reminding people of my disability, as though I were some little kid who had to keep crying in order to get food. I did want to talk about other things besides my limitations. But when people in my life said or did things that showed their lack of memory and respect, I felt like I had to bring it up again. Then, I felt self-conscious because I was bringing so much attention to my disability. It was a Catch 22 situation, and in either case, I felt unappreciated.

Even medical professionals don't get it

Non-medically trained people in my life didn't understand my predicament, but I didn't think I'd get the same lack of understanding from people who had studied medicine. I was wrong again!

I had been seen by many of the strabismus experts in the Bay Area and none of them had ever told me I couldn't see in 3D. I had to discover that via Dr. Oliver Sacks' magazine article. Even eye doctors weren't disclosing to patients the impact a lack of binocular vision could have. I wondered how many kids with binocular vision issues didn't understand why they had trouble with team sports like basketball, where hand-eye coordination is key.

One warm February afternoon in California, I met my friend at a restaurant in Mountain View, right across from the train station. He and I had spoken about my issue many times before. He was a gastroenterologist, so obviously his specialty was the stomach and not the eyes. But he had a very close friend who was an ophthalmologist, with whom he had discussed my situation. I was telling him about the Dalí painting and about how happy I was to see diplopia depicted on the canvas, he looked at me puzzled, furrowed his brows and said, "Wait, but you don't have double vision."

"I've been talking to you about my double vision for a long time," I responded.

Inside, I was very upset. I didn't announce to him every time I saw him in double or had diplopia but we had discussed double vision.

This wasn't the first time that I had spoken to a medical professional whom I knew personally who didn't know that somebody with my condition could see in double. Didn't they study this in medical school? We make up about three percent of the population. Wasn't there at least a paragraph about us in medical textbooks stating that people who have asymmetric eyes could see in double?

Perhaps for this friend, because he hadn't been in a medical school classroom for a few decades, that paragraph which he had once read many years ago had disappeared from his memory.

It was moments like these that really made me take pause about how much I wanted to share. I hoped that people with a medical background who were well meaning could understand the context of what I was discussing, but I was wrong about that too—they still couldn't remember or understand.

Further fueling this disenchantment was a BBC podcast called *The Power of the Image* with a Harvard Medical School professor, Dr. Margaret Livingstone. The Harvard Medical School neurobiologist explained that not seeing depth well could be an asset to artists. But, when asked about how stereoblind people survive in life without binocular vision, she said that monocular people made more use of monocular depth cues than binocular people and didn't experience a deficit. According to her stereoblind friend, they only had minor problems, like not being able to thread a needle easily.

I was infuriated. Not having 3D vision was not just about not being able to thread a needle well! I doubt Dr. Livingstone intended to de-legitimize our plight, but she made our problems seem elementary. Beyond the driving, parking and sports issues, some people have major difficulties reading that got them stuck in remedial classes in school because their ophthalmologists didn't refer them to vision therapy to remedy their eye coordination problems. If threading a needle were the worst of our problems, then many more of us would drive, few of the developmental optometrists would have a job, and no one would bother with vision therapy to gain 3D.

Dr. Margaret Livingstone's words could make a HUGE impact on medicine. She taught at one of the most prestigious medical institutions in the world and her students could turn out to be like the ophthalmologists many of us have dealt with who didn't even bother to tell us that we can't see in 3D. These doctors might not see it as a problem and therefore won't refer their patients to vision therapy or, in the case of children, tell the child's parents about the problems associated with being stereo-blind.

I wrote Dr. Livingstone a letter explaining how her comments belittled our struggles as patients and the work of vision therapists and developmental optometrists. She never responded.

As I got more and more frustrated with not being able to discuss amblyopia with people in my life because they couldn't understand me, I sought out professional help from psychologists. What was even more shocking than doctors or a neurobiologist being ignorant was when I consulted psychological counselors who were clueless. None of them had ever heard of the impact of binocular visual disorders! It was more aggravating for me to have to pay psychologists while educating them on my condition than it was for me to just keep my mouth shut.

Driving

I am driving my parents to my ten-year-old nephew's birthday party. We are on Bascom Avenue in San Jose, California and I see the restaurant on the left side of the street. To turn left into the restaurant, I have to take an unprotected left turn on a major thoroughfare with several lanes of traffic coming my way. Skipping the unprotected left turn, I drive a couple more blocks and make a U-Turn at the next stoplight and then go back to the street with the restaurant.

"Why, why did you stop? Why did you skip that street? There, there's the restaurant right there," my dad yells out when I pass the restaurant.

"I know, but it's too uncomfortable for me to make the left turn here so I'm going to go to the light," I respond.

Then my mom, who didn't hear me explain it to my father, asks me the same question.

"It's hard for me to judge the distance of these cars and how fast they're going. It's easier for me to drive two more blocks and make a protected U-turn when I have no oncoming traffic," I explain.

"Well, I've been to this restaurant before and I always just turn left here," my Mom responds.

I take a deep breath. I don't want to get into an argument while I'm in the driver's seat because that could make the situation even more difficult. I had told my parents many times how difficult it was for me to drive and how people with my condition have trouble judging distance. They still don't understand why I choose the longer road, which is safer.

We get to the restaurant. There is only one cook working for the whole restaurant. We have to wait a long time for the food and we are all hungry. My strabismic aunt Lila joins us.

"Do you skip unprotected left turns and wait until you can get to the next stoplight and make a U-turn?" I ask.

"Yes, of course. I can't make unprotected left turns. It's too unsafe for me because I can't see how fast the traffic is going," she says.

I turn to my parents and say, "Look, this is another example of somebody who does this. It's not that I'm crazy."

This was one of many situations I had over the years while driving. Sometimes I'd pass a very small parallel parking spot on a street, and I'd keep driving down the street and even go to another street, until I could find a parking spot that had more space. Inevitably whoever was in the car with me would say, "Why did you skip that spot? I would have parked there. You can make it." I had to explain, "Well, it's very hard for me. I'd rather walk two extra blocks to get to where I need to go than park in an area that's too difficult for me."

Even now, I still have to repark my car in front of my house when the vehicle is too far from the curb. I would have thought that after all of these years of parking in the same place, I would have learned to do it right, but alas, that is not the case.

Sometimes when I had to merge into the right lane quickly in order to turn onto a street or get off the highway, my heart would beat faster and I was afraid. I missed exits on the highway because I couldn't merge fast enough. I would get off at another exit, go back a stop on the highway or take surface streets to get to where I wanted to go.

When I saw a car merging on the right of the freeway, it looked like it was coming very close, my heart started to beat really fast or it skipped a beat and I got scared of causing an accident.

I'd even take a circumvented route to get to my own home. If somebody was in my car, they could think that I'd forgotten how to get to my house! I preferred to be late, use more fuel and annoy the person in the car with me than possibly cause an accident.

One of my aunts who is strabismic didn't take the highway at all because of all the stress. She felt like cars were coming right towards her. She navigated only surface streets, which meant that a drive that could take me 20 minutes on the highway could take her 45 minutes or an hour taking various surface roads.

This inconvenience to one's daily life because of driving is not miniscule. Unless one is living in a big city like New York or Chicago where one doesn't need a car, most places in the United States require the use of a vehicle. I know an amblyope who moved to San Francisco precisely so that he wouldn't have to drive.

Some well-wishers sometimes suggested, "If it's so hard for you to drive, why don't you just move to a big city?", ignoring that rents could be much higher in a big city. Maybe I wouldn't have the same social circle there or have the same job opportunities. It is very easy to give this blanket prescription, along the lines of horse manure advice. Not everyone can drop their life and move to a metropolis with good public transportation, just like not everyone with allergies can move to the desert.

The Need for Connection

Like an immigrant to a new land, I longed for people who understood me. Immigrants often gravitated to people from their same country or language group so that they could have people to talk to who understood what it was like to be in between countries, cultures and language groups. Their families back home may not have understood the cultural problems they had in their new country. Friends made in their new country could be ignorant of what their lives were like back home and why they struggled so much with culture shock and new ways of doing things in their adopted country.

I had only a handful of people online and in real life who had been in between 2D and 3D. I was like an immigrant or refugee from a country no one had ever heard of. Trying to explain the culture and habitat of my world was like a Martian telling us what life is like on Mars.

Some friends and family members were surprised that I suddenly had this newfound desire, if not passion, to meet other people who had my condition and talk to them about their vision and how it had affected them. "Well, you've never talked about this before. Why are you suddenly so interested in it?" Others even posited that if I hadn't read that article by Oliver Sacks, my life would have been better. I would not have known about lacking 3D vision.

The reason I had rarely talked about my situation with my eyes was because I had few people with whom to discuss it. When I saw people on the street, at the library or wherever with noticeably divergent eyes or an eye patch, I automatically wanted to speak to them and connect, but I didn't want to make these strangers feel uncomfortable. Even with people who weren't complete strangers to me, I also had to be careful. Before I read about Sue Barry, I encountered only a couple of people I wanted to talk with about the eye problems we seemed to share.

In 1998 I had a dinner at an Italian restaurant in downtown Sunnyvale with colleagues for a birthday celebration. Louisa, one of my colleagues, had brought her brother who had a noticeably wandering eye. I didn't want to put him on the spot at the dinner. But after the dinner, I spoke to Louisa in private.

"Louisa, your brother and I, we have the same condition," I said.

"What? What are you talking about?" Louisa said.

"Our eyes. I also have amblyopia."

"But your eyes look straight."

"They do now. I've had two operations but I'm still an amblyope and I have strabismus like your brother. Let him know that he can talk to me."

Her brother never spoke to me. I never brought up the topic again. I knew that it could be extremely uncomfortable for people, and I didn't want to call attention to someone's eyes, especially in front of others.

A couple of years later when I was living in San Francisco, my roommate was a mentor to a young Hispanic girl. When this girl came over to our apartment, I immediately saw that both of her eyes were asymmetric. I didn't say anything, not wanting to put her on the spot. She had a lot of energy and was very talkative. We talked about other things that were happening in her life and school. When the girl left, I spoke to my roommate about her.

"You know, if your mentee ever wants to talk about her eye condition, I'm here. I've had those operations myself."

Carolina looked at me just like Louisa had and said, "What are you talking about?" I explained to her that I also was strabismic. The girl never approached me to talk about the operation.

In 2013, I was on a plane from Frankfurt to San Francisco. The woman sitting next to me was an American living in Paris. We talked about various subjects, including her late husband, and gospel music in Paris. Somehow, we got onto the topic of our vision. I didn't usually open up to just anybody about my eyes. I told her I did vision therapy.

"Oh, my gosh. I've never spoken to anybody else with this condition," she said.

"What?" I said, surprised.

"I'm an amblyope, too, and I also went to UC Berkeley to do vision therapy as a child. I did patching. Nothing helped and I stopped."

She had never spoken to anybody who knew about the condition. Like with my case, her eyes appeared to be symmetric. She just kept quiet her whole life. Sometimes her late husband wouldn't understand when they went rock climbing and she had difficulty judging distances. This woman was old enough to be my mother and she went through her entire life without being able to share anything about her situation.

When I met people on the Internet with 2D vision, I felt this great sense of camaraderie. We'd say to each other, "You understand what I'm going through. Can you give me tips? What do I do when people keep forgetting my limitations?" I wished I had those people next to me, to go on walks with so we could both look at trees together and talk about how our vision was changing. We could look at water droplets on open cucumbers and talk about how beautiful it was. I didn't want to always have to do this on my own and describe it by using computer keystrokes. I wanted to be able to revel in this new world with people around me who could tell me about what they saw that I hadn't seen yet.

Through the Internet, I met another woman who was going through vision therapy at UC Berkeley. We met one day by Peet's Coffee on Shattuck Avenue by the Downtown Berkeley BART station. We went for a walk on campus and we stopped by a tree and I said, "Tell me: what do you see when you look at this tree and you rock back and forth?" She described to me how she saw the distance between branches. "Wow, this is what I've been longing for. Standing under a tree, rocking back and forth like a child, with somebody else who understands what I'm going through," I thought. She told me about how when she walked outside her door, she saw more distance between her neighbors' homes and the trees in front of their homes. That's a distance she never saw before. She understood my social isolation. She told me she had lost most of her friends because they didn't understand what was going on with her, even though she had been there for them when they were experiencing troubling times. In some respects, her side effects were worse than mine.

I felt calmed. Somebody else was also going through this and could empathize. She knew what it was like to live in a world that was hard to describe to other people in a way that they could understand. I met her a couple of times but she didn't live nearby. We couldn't go on regular walks together and stare at plants and talk about how it looked like the plants were coming towards us.

It was like I needed a playmate or a jungle gym with other kids. Until I became a research subject in the lab, I returned to my childhood by doing vision therapy but I didn't have a playpen where there were other kids. I couldn't go to the playground and swing on the swings with other kids and talk about how the trees looked different when we were moving back and forth or compare how the trees looked different now than they did before VT and describe how the branches were coming towards us. I had to live in my own world, be my own best friend, my own playmate. Other people I had met on the Internet who were going through vision therapy and had seen their worlds change also shared this sense of isolation.

Empathy

I found that as I had been going through this whole process of realizing my limitations and becoming my own companion and also realizing where I had to censor myself, I had developed a much stronger form of empathy for people who had lived in repression their whole lives. Whether it was that they had to hide their political beliefs, religion or sexuality, not being able to say what one truly felt generated an immense amount of tension, stress, grief and guilt.

I thought about people who, for example, were gay and were living in a homophobic society, and had to attend family events and hear family members say homophobic remarks. Or somebody of a particular religion living in a country where they couldn't exercise their faith, forced to practice in secret while listening to pejorative comments at school, the workplace and with their family members. They couldn't tell people what they really believed in, what their thoughts were, why they didn't eat certain foods and why they didn't do certain activities.

Having worked on various elections in former communist countries, I knew of activists who had worked on their causes when it was very dangerous to stand up for one's beliefs. They could have been jailed, sent to a camp for political prisoners during Soviet times or be killed. These people took immense risks to be who they were but they had to do it in secret.

Although my issue with asymmetric eyes and sensitivity to noise was minuscule in comparison to people who had to risk their lives for personal or political reasons, I could empathize with what it was like to conceal one's true self and have to be in situations that were extremely uncomfortable and could gnaw away at one's integrity.

It was this exact empathy that I was missing from many of my friends who tried to be there in their own way to help me, but couldn't empathize.

Socially unacceptable

As driving was often a problem for me, I was grateful for those who offered me a ride when I needed one. However, turning down rides could be difficult. Getting a ride to an event meant that I had to talk to the driver for the entire time I was in the car, when actually, what I really needed was silence. Sometimes it was actually preferable for me to drive to an event, even if it was at night, so that I could drive in silence and have the mental clarity I needed.

This became really uncomfortable for me to explain to people, "You know, thanks for offering me a ride but actually, I'd prefer for you not to talk to me." People would be offended and not understand. I would have to make up excuses or find some way to get to an event without offending other people.

I always had to think of a Plan B for social events. Months before attending a good friend's wedding, I was already thinking, "What do I do if it's too loud at the wedding? Am I going to leave and possibly offend the bride and the groom? The wedding is four hours away by car. Do I carpool with people, save money, and be in a car with four other people talking the whole time? Do I share a house with ten people and a dog? Do I drive on my own, be in silence, stay in a place on my own and pay up to four times more than if I were to share with others?" But when I didn't think of finances and I put my mental health first, I realized that even though it was hard for me to drive, it was better for me to drive on my own so that I could have mental clarity and silence and be completely present at the wedding.

Usually people go to weddings and are happy. They dance and drink. The day after driving several hours on my own on the windy coastal Californian highway, I barely drank at the wedding. I didn't dance because it was too loud inside and I spent most of my time outside, sometimes walking around the pumpkin patch or in the parking lot by myself because the loud music was too much for me.

My friend Savannah, one of the people who encouraged me to do VT, told me the same thing about needing an exit strategy for social events where she might get overwhelmed and her vision might become unstable.

One of the positive side effects of VT was that I learned to put my health before money.

Comparative silliness

What was also difficult socially was to rejoice in my new vision with those around me.

"Why is it that you felt like you were a freak when you talked about dust and flies?" my editor, who is also an amblyope, asked me.

"How many other adults in their 30s talk about their fascination with moisture on a cucumber? Usually the only people that I've ever heard of who speak like that are people who are on psychedelic drugs, who find the crevices in an orange peel to be beyond fascinating," I responded.

I wasn't taking mind-altering substances nor did I want others to think I was doing drugs. I wanted people to appreciate what I was going through, but I felt extremely self-conscious talking about it because what I was seeing seemed trivial. I had also told my friends about how expensive this therapy was. What was difficult to explain was that it wasn't just the cucumbers, flies and snow that I was happy about, but also the skills to see better with both of my eyes. If someone did a Return on Investment (ROI) analysis on the money I spent on VT and the benefits I received: flies, snow, mildew and moisture on cucumbers, they wouldn't see the value.

After about three years in therapy, I called a friend to congratulate him on the birth of his second child. He had recently received venture capital funding for his cloud computing business to the tune of $22 million. He had an office with a view of the San Francisco Bay in the very expensive Transamerica Tower in San Francisco. He had bought a pricey home in Marin County, a yacht, drove a German SUV from Marin County to

San Francisco for work, had an apartment in Paris and traveled around the world for his business. When he asked me how I was doing, I was too embarrassed to tell him about my flies. I actually thought that where he was, in this skyscraper in San Francisco, he probably didn't even see white flies that high up. However, he might be able to see dust coming in through the window. Especially to somebody like him, a financial investor, I felt too silly to talk about how my vision was changing.

When my friend in Miami called me to tell me about her new gorgeous Italian boyfriend, I didn't want to tell her that my visual acuity had improved so much that I could see mildew, the same thing that people usually want to scrape out of their shower and not have to see, with or without glasses. How could my mildew and mold in the shower compare with her Italian hunk?

Comparing my VT victories to what was happening in the lives of my friends caused me to withdraw. Even though not everybody in my life everyday had a new Adonis-esque Italian boyfriend or had struck gold in the lottery of Silicon Valley venture capital funding, I still felt that sharing my struggles and my victories with dust, mist, flies and mildew seemed miniscule and childish. I stopped calling people to ask how they were doing because I realized that I most likely would not want to share what was happening with me because people wouldn't understand or they would laugh.

As I communicated with more people with 2D vision and VT patients on the Internet, I realized that they shared my social problems. One of my inspirations to publish this book was that if I talked about the struggles that I had gone through in VT, I could help others at least understand the context of the victories of people in VT. Obviously a $22 million investment in a company is huge, but for another person, seeing the moisture on a cut cucumber for the first time can also be a major victory.

We can't live and speak only in specialized websites and Internet chat rooms

After reading the book *Living Well with a Hidden Disability*, I learned that people who have other hidden disabilities—whatever they are, whether it's a sleeping disability or another disability yet-to-be discussed on *The Doctors* TV show—faced the same troubles I did.

At the same time I struggled to have others understand what I was speaking about, I wanted them to understand that just because I saw in 2D didn't mean my life wasn't rich. Just like somebody who has autism processes information differently, it didn't mean that they couldn't enjoy music and other joys. Their brains just work in a different way.

If we as a society could grow to accept or at least be aware of the fact that there are various ways of processing visual, auditory, tactile and other inputs, then it would be easier for all of us who don't have common ways of being or typical appearances to feel more comfortable about ourselves and not be relegated to only discussing our lives in separate Internet chat rooms. If we turn into a society where only people with eye problems can discuss their vision together and only people with hearing problems can discuss their auditory issues in special Yahoo or Google Groups, we're not actually hearing each other. We're not seeing each other. We're just becoming a segregated world based on self-interests. That doesn't lead to a richer society. That just leads to people feeling isolated, and that's exactly how I felt throughout this whole process of trying to see like others. A world of conversations in silos leads to more silos.

Not all VT patients will react the way I did. Not all family members and friends will make the same mistakes of inviting VT patients to events they can't attend, bugging them about driving, giving unsolicited advice and telling them to stop improving their vision. My stories are cautions, not directions.

If you have limited depth perception or are doing VT, be warned that despite your efforts to the contrary, some people will never understand you. Know your audience.

If you have a friend with binocular vision problems, do your best to remember your friend's limitations and main concerns, even if you don't understand.

If reading this chapter can help prevent heartaches, both on the side of the VT patient and their friends and family, then the time I took to write this book has been validated.

I hope you won't suffer as much as I did. Or hopefully, not at all.

Please see the tips in Chapter Six for both VT patients and those supporting them for suggestions on how to handle social invitations, conversations about VT, and other health-related matters.

Growing frustrated with his dance protegé, the Argentine tango expert, Pablo Veron, keeps telling his student, Sally Potter:

"Il faut trouver ton axe." (You have to find your center.)

"Tenés* que encontrar tu eje." (You have to find your center.)

In the movie "The Tango Lesson," Sally Potter plays herself, a British filmmaker, who is learning to dance tango with the famous Pablo Veron. The dialogue in the movie alternates between French, Spanish and English.

Veron is telling Potter she needs to find her center and then she can dance. Otherwise, she could dance off-beat, be confused and frustrate her dance partner.

These phrases about finding my center ring in my ears when the doctor tells me I am seeing things in two places because my brain has two right answers for everything. I have two different places to center my eyes, the old way and the new way.

Voy a encontrar mi eje. Je vais trouver mon axe. I will find my center.

And then, and only then, will I twirl.

*Tenés is the Argentine vos form of the second person singular. Most Spanish speakers would say "tienes" and not "tenés"

– CHAPTER FIVE –

Changing Vision ⇒ Changing Life

Throughout my time doing vision therapy, I realized that I was not only opening up my brain to stop suppressing my vision, but I was centering myself and my vision and becoming aware of suppressed emotions. I had to slow down, radically change my social calendar or eliminate it completely and be more selective about the people I let into my life. The small things, like flying dust and mildew, became a constant source of wonder for me, almost an escape from the side effects and isolation I felt from changing my brain.

My friend Liz correctly pointed out that I was going through the stages of grief. At first, I didn't understand what she meant since no one had died and I hadn't lost anything. She told me I had lost the dream of dramatically improving my depth perception and completing the bulk of VT in a year. (VT is never over. A patient still has to do exercises to maintain what they have gained.) The five stages of grief, according to Elizabeth Kubler-Ross, are: denial, anger, depression bargaining and acceptance. I don't think I ever experienced the bargaining stage. But the first step was being in denial that I had a veritable disability. I became angry and depressed that my life was changing quickly but my progress was slow. I couldn't go out at night and my friends didn't understand me. Once I moved into acceptance, life became much easier and smoother.

Vacillating: making decisions to stay stable

Parallel to my eyes finding and staying at the right answer, I wanted to find my center.

I wondered if my vacillating between the right place for my eyes and the old or wrong place was correlated to my own life. I knew I shouldn't be getting attached to a traveling Brazilian who said he couldn't commit to a relationship, but I let myself get close to him even though I knew it wasn't a wise idea. It's like I knew what my eyes should be seeing and sometimes I saw what I was supposed to see and sometimes I didn't. Could putting my foot down and saying "no" to the traveling and poorly communicative *brasileiro* at all affect my stability in life and perhaps the stabilization of my vision?

I used to be like the Brazilian, traveling all the time and not always available to be in a relationship, at times too tired to email or call when traveling for work. But I was not that person anymore, nor did I want to be. Due to the therapy, I couldn't travel that much and I craved stability.

I wanted to stabilize to the right place where I should be seeing with both eyes and not to the old (incorrect) place. My goal was to develop depth perception and to have stability in my personal life. Could I get to depth and stability if I consciously vacillated between incorrect and correct ways of being? Perhaps "correct" wasn't the right word for my way of being, but I could take steps that would be more conducive to getting on the road to what I wanted.

My vision therapy was more like brain therapy rather than eye therapy because most of the changes were happening in my brain, not in my eyes. The idea that a change in my thinking about my life could affect my vision was not such a far cry from reality. Once my brain accepted Point B as my new way of seeing the world, then I was advancing with my therapy. But if I had one foot in the door of Point B, but still felt magnetized to Point A, I was screwing up my therapy. Point A was no longer where I wanted to be. I dedicated myself to this therapy because I wanted to be at Point B and all other points that led to 3D.

My changing abilities with the red-green letter and number chart was an example of having two "right" answers. The color chart exercise became harder to do and I saw more in double. The optometrist explained that this was a good thing because I was breaking the suppression and abnormal retinal correspondence (ARC). It was so counter-intuitive that an exercise becoming more difficult was actually a good sign. One would think that an exercise should get easier the more one does it, but actually it was the opposite. Initially, when wearing the red-green glasses, I could see the letters in the colored (green and red) boxes without a problem. The goal of looking at the Hart Chart with red-green glasses was to make sure I was using both

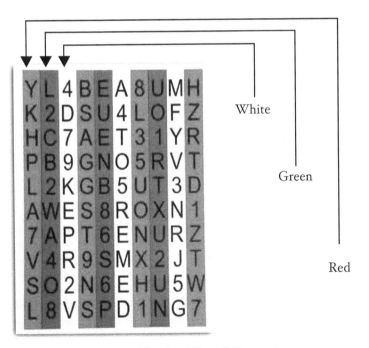

Red-Green Hart Chart™, ©Bernell Corporation

eyes. If I could see all of the columns, then my brain was using both of my eyes.

The more I did the exercise, the harder it was to see the letters in their boxes without seeing in double. I saw the letter in one place and the box in another. This was a good thing because my anomalous retinal correspondence was giving me the "right" answer, while my eyes were both vertically and horizontally misaligned because my brain was telling me what the picture "should" look like rather than how my eyes actually saw it. When my brain wasn't trying to make the picture perfect, I saw the letters and the boxes horizontally and vertically misaligned and in double.

VT ⇒ Knowing myself

Becoming aware of my reasons for doing certain things was quite eye-opening. It wasn't until 2008 when my yoga teacher told me I was tilting my head that I realized I had been tilting my head most of my life, unconsciously. Then I noticed that one of my strabismic aunts did it too. When I met Savannah, my teacher friend who had done VT for suppression and convergence issues, she noticed that I often tilted my head and blinked. Since our eyes are not straight, a slight repositioning of the head could bring us to a posture where we can see straight and avoid double vision. Savannah posited that I was blinking a lot to avoid double vision and suppression.

By learning about my many difficulties, I discovered aspects about my habitual behaviors. While walking with my friend Medie on an uneven sidewalk, I couldn't look at her from the side because I always had my head pointed towards the ground to make sure I wouldn't trip or fall over the breaks in the concrete. Over a year later, I fell and sprained my ankle while walking at night in Sarajevo. There was a pothole in the street that was probably made by a bomb during the 1992-1996 war. I emailed Medie about my fall and she responded, "I understand clearly now why you were particular about where we took our walks. To add to things I take for granted: depth perception." Some of my falls and ankle sprains were directly tied to my not seeing well when walking on uneven ground.

Medie was a fan of tide pooling. One time I joined her and other friends on the beach to see the sea creatures in low-tide. While others quickly ascended the rocks, I wasn't aware of what exactly I was calculating in my mind when deciding where to step, but I walked very slowly and deliberately on the slippery rocks. It took me much longer to assess where I could step because I was analyzing which rocks shone less and were therefore less wet and slippery. I didn't climb up wet rocks on a daily basis, but these types of activities, which to others are second nature and require no conscious thought, can slow down those of us in 2D land. Just like for many years I didn't understand why merging traffic and parking were so troubling for me, uncovering the reasons behind my slow walking or extra caution was comforting.

Altering one's view of the world will fundamentally modify how one behaves and interacts. I had no idea my life would change as much as it did and is still changing. Some experience these awakenings or illuminations via religious or spiritual pursuits; mine came by rewiring my brain.

Taking a break, to return to myself!

After eight months in VT, I asked my developmental optometrist if I could take a break from VT. I told him that I needed to recharge my batteries and maybe even travel.

My first few weeks without VT were blissful. I wanted to go back to being my vibrant self. Just returning to being the energetic person whom I'd always known myself to be was such a gift. I didn't need jewelry, money or clothes. I just wanted to be myself. A friend of mine who had gone through cancer treatment completely understood my sentiment as he was also happy to just be normal again.

I almost felt like the sleeping sickness patients in the movie *Awakenings*, who rejoiced at going dancing or seeing girls in short skirts after so many years of being dormant. Granted, my situation wasn't nearly as extreme as those who were in a state of sleep for decades, but for a super energetic person like myself to be resigned to only reading and staying at home, returning to myself was a treat. I did know, of course, that when I resumed therapy after a month or so, I would come back to my headaches, fatigue, confusion and need for silence. I didn't care. I wanted to enjoy every second of being alive, being vibrant and spending time with friends.

Surrendering to being a new person

After a month or so of my break, I went right back to VT feeling refreshed and energetic.

Around Thanksgiving in 2010, I reveled in my quiet time. I stayed at home and watched movies and met with friends. While talking to my Spanish friend Marilo, I told her that I was letting go of trying to be who I used to be before vision therapy. She said, "You're preparing now for who you will be after your therapy is over." She was right. Clinging to the past was not only not serving me, it was pointless. I was evolving and aging and it was to be expected that I would transform over time. It just happened that in 2010, as a result of my fatigue, concentration problems and other VT side effects, a lot of change occurred in a short period of time and with an unexpected frequency.

Like in the biblical story of Lot's wife, I realized there was no point in looking back. I wouldn't turn into a pillar of salt, but looking back to try to be who I was before was only going to bring salty tears and make my life worse.

I was surrendering myself to the process and I stopped trying to control where I was going or to understand what was going on. Surrendering was not giving up: it was about giving up control. I imagined that this might be one of the biggest hurdles for an adult doing VT. The type of person attracted to voluntarily do VT (not due to an immediate need for therapy because of their eyes being unstable), who was willing to make the financial, health, social and other sacrifices, was most likely a high achieving risk-taker. Usually those who were so determined to make major leaps preferred to be in control because otherwise, it was like crossing a threshold blindfolded, not knowing where the path was going. Without any intended pun, doing VT for someone who was stereo-blind was like going into a new road blindfolded and having to trust the process with few signposts or people to help along the way. This required a profound mental leap of faith.

Sue Barry and my friend Savannah both did vision therapy out of necessity because their vision was breaking down. That was not my situation.

Once I surrendered myself to VT, my life actually became easier. I felt less friction deciding between how I used to do things and leading my life in a new, less active way. But I would not have been able to surrender on Day 1 of VT. I had to go through the energy swings, intermittent double vision and sights of small wonders like orange peel texture to give myself up and see and feel life anew.

New Vision of Life

One evening, my friend Elisa came over for dinner and I was telling her about how I felt like I was at a crossroads in my life, although I was not sure where the roads in front of me would lead. All I knew was that the charted paths behind me must stay in the past. I couldn't be the person I was before because I simply didn't have the energy to be as social.

I also told her that I had been resisting the temptation to call certain people who would most likely complain to me about their lives, as I was having enough of my own issues.

It seemed selfish, but I realized I wasn't being selfish. I was being smart. I needed to focus on myself.

"So your vision therapy is literally giving you a clearer perspective on your life," Elisa said.

Yes, indeed. As more and more things came into my visual field, I was examining my life and seeing what it was that I wanted to keep in my horizon and what had to go.

I re-read the following reader's comments several times throughout my VT journey, as these observations helped me find the courage to focus on myself and spend less time solving other people's problems.

Commenter #14:

Hey there, Princess,

When I was a 37-year-old single mom of two young boys, I lost my vision completely. Within minutes, a rare auto-immune disorder took me from 20/20 vision to nothing at all. Originally, doctors at Stanford predicted I would lose everything within a year. Today, I have no light perception (NLP) on my left eye.

But I have vision in my right eye that fluctuates between 20/70 and 2200. I truly believe the work I've done with my brain and my thinking has helped improve my vision.

So you hang in there. We're all rootin' for you!

Trite as this is going to sound, losing my vision was the first step in truly seeing my life. Not only where it was, but where I wanted to go. And it gave me the clarity (once I was over the rage) to put my priorities and values in order.

It takes a tremendous amount of physical and mental energy to do the kind of vision therapy you are doing. Only a few of my friends really understood when I was too exhausted to lend a good listening ear, to meet for lunch, or even a simple cup of coffee. I learned to rely on those friends who DID understand...understand, for example, the test of dressing so you look at least somewhat put together, getting out of your house, crossing a threshold into a restaurant or coffee house that is unfamiliar. I mean that stuff is paralyzingly scary to me. And scary ultimately equals drained.

When I was doing intense mental work to restore at least partial vision, I found it to be a time for me to lovingly, kindly explain to all my friends that my focus had to be on my sight, not on them. There were those who got huffy and "fired" me. As much as it hurt at the time, I was relieved to know who was really in my corner. I was relieved that I no longer had to be a shoulder to my friends when I had barely a shoulder for myself.

Sounds cold, but it's a time for a certain amount of brutality. **When you are through this, THEN you can be of help to others.**

You are handling this situation with wisdom and a curious eye. No pun intended. It sounds like you are doing great. And if Elisa is willing... then she's about the best friend you could have right now. She sounds blessedly intuitive and compassionate.

The commenter was right. Once I went through the hurdles of VT, I could write this book to help others.

Law of Attraction and vision therapy: How to envision 3D when you can only see in 2D

In 2011, I joined Sovoto: The Vision Advocacy Network, an on-line community for those doing VT, parents of VT patients and VT practitioners. (See the Resources section for the website address.) I posed the following question in the forum for Adult Strabismics about how someone in my position could imagine what 3D would be like.

I'm 15 months in VT aiming to see in 3D and I need some psychological encouragement. For those who are not into "New Age" thought, this may seem esoteric to you, but the power of the mind is vast and I want to use positive thinking to get me to seeing with both eyes and fusing.

I'm reading the book "Power" by Rhonda Byrne. It's the sequel to the international bestseller, "The Secret" which was also an Internet movie hit. For those not familiar with "The Secret" and the "Law of Attraction," the basic premise is that to bring something into one's life, one has to imagine that he/she already has it, feel that he/she has it and believe that he/she has it. "Like attracts like" so you have to be on the same vibration of what you want in order for it to come to you. If you want a new car, you imagine what it looks like, you feel what it's like to drive it and you believe you really own it. Thinking about not having something, like I do about 3D, is not getting me closer to having stereopsis because it only makes me more anxious, frustrated, etc.

Visualization is a key tool for the law of attraction, but those of us who are stereoblind can't visualize something to which we are blind. So we need help, or at least I do.

Here's my question to optometrists and to anyone who has crossed the bridge from flatland to binocularity: how does it feel to see in 3D as opposed to 2D? I am not asking what it looks like because that's too abstract for me. People describe depth and they might as well be speaking in Greek; I don't understand anything. I am not talking about the feelings of surprise at the steering wheel popping out or the cherry tomato in the lunch salad popping (examples from "Fixing My Gaze"), but what does it feel like to see in 3D?

I want to feel what it's like to see in 3D to help me get there, but my only experience was with 3D glasses looking at a computer screen and seeing the soccer ball come out of the screen. I can't transpose that experience to the real world because it's freaky to imagine everything popping out of where it is and I have no idea how to do that.

Here is the answer I came up with after reading some excellent responses from a developmental optometrist and other amblyopes who had crossed over from 2D to 3D.

Note to myself as though I were writing to a friend:

I thought about what it might feel like to see in 3D and I inquired with those on the other side of the binocular road and learned that they feel more comfortable when they see in 3D because they know their distance from objects around them. When I do see positive changes in my vision (not like the times I saw friends with two heads), I'm in awe. What I keep in my mind and heart is a sense of awe to the world. This has been HUGE! I am in a better mood and more positive.

APRIL 25:

I've been enjoying looking at the rain and raindrops on roses. When I'd seen photos of raindrops on flowers before, they had seemed too beautiful to be real. It had never occured to me that people could actually see rain drops on flowers in such detail until I saw them myself. Whereas I used to think that the raindrops had been altered on a computer, now I see that it's my brain and eyes that are being altered.

MAY 5:

I went for a nice evening springtime walk today and was admiring nature. It felt as though the trees, plants and flowers were moving towards me as I walked to them. But inanimate things like cars and houses stood still. Yesterday, the carpet on the gym floor was of special interest. Today, as I was raking the small wisteria leaves from the patio and putting them into the yard waste can, I was remarking at how cool it was to see the ray of sun cast light on the leaves as they fell into the can. The less I think of the side effects (like sleeping 10 plus hours last night) and the more I concentrate on the simple beauty of my new world of approaching trees and flowers, the happier I am.

Commenter #8 says:

Susanna, obviously I can't tell you what it feels like to see in 3D, being wildly strabismic, but I can tell you the feeling I get from using the Brock string successfully. When I see "out of the center of my head," that is, when I see with both eyes equally, albeit at 3" or 4" (7.6-10 cm), I get a warm feeling in the center of my chest. It feels like something has opened up.

As far as visualizing being New Age, well, maybe it is these days, but my father, now 98 years old and hardly a stereotypical guru (picturing a successful cowboy wouldn't be too far off the mark) would always tell me to picture what I'd want, that getting the picture right was the important part of any job. I saw it work for him time and time again, and in the most improbable situations, from laying pipe to finding stolen bicycles to buying his ranch.

The inner voyage to create distance in my life and vision, *La fine è il mio inizio* (The end is my beginning)

A few years before doing VT, I immersed myself into two huge books in Italian about the end of the life of the Italian journalist, Tiziano Terzani. As he was dying from cancer, he sat down with his son and told him about some of his trajectory from growing up in a poor family in Florence after World War II. Terzani had won scholarships to study in New York and China and worked as a reporter in Asia.

While in VT, I realized the parallels in our lives. I was also a writer, a globetrotter and I was on the most difficult journey ever, one for which I had no passport, visa, map, guide or internal compass to guide me. The road to stereovision forced me to accept an inner journey through my mind.

Terzani was at peace with himself. His longing to travel and explore went away as he journeyed further inside himself because of his cancer. He gave up meat and ate simply, adoring his quiet time admiring the sunsets in the Himalayas and Orsigna, Italy.

I watched an interview Terzani gave soon before he died. He smiled when he said that having cancer gave him an excellent excuse to avoid going to stuffy social events he didn't want to attend, ambassador's receptions, and the like. Instead of meeting with acquaintances and friends to hear about the news in their lives, he dedicated himself to his meditation, walks and travel. He had done chemotherapy, homeopathy and many different types of alternative care but nothing worked. He seemed quite happy in the interview, stating that he realized that there would never be a cure for his cancer and that the only person who could make him feel better was himself.

Luckily my drive to improve my vision didn't come from a fear of death, it came from a genuine desire to see more of life. Similar to Terzani, my need for isolation and silence were positive side effects and I was grateful to have an excuse to be selective with my time.

I became more and more content with the free time I had created in my life as I cut out many activities to make room for my vision therapy and resulting fatigue.

At first, I resented the fact that I wasn't able to do as many activities as before and be with friends, and then I reveled in my quiet. For the first time in my life, I had zero plans. My life turned into an open slate and I loved it!

As I was training my brain to see space, I was creating space in my life, so much so that I grew to be happy with the nothingness of a grand expanse of time and space before me, virgin territory on which I could paint my new life.

When I was a kid and having fun "moving objects with my eyes," and seeing small colors move on my white walls and ceiling, I was happily inhabiting a magical world alone. As an adult, I wanted to make sense of the magical world and find words to explain it to myself and others. I realized that those vibrating colors on my white walls were probably due to my eyes quickly alternating and my brain picking up on reflections of lights and vibrations. But who in my adult world would understand that I could still see walls vibrate? Once I realized how incredibly fortunate I was to become a child again and be astonished by the simple beauties of seeing the rain and snow clearly, I went back to living in an enchanted forest, filled with wonder and delight. And I didn't have to share it with anyone! This realization was a major breakthrough as I stepped out of the confines of explanation and words that define adult life.

La terapia visiva è il mio inizio. (Vision therapy is my beginning).

How many second opinions can a girl have?

As my life turned upside down, I sought more professional expertise. I counted how many health professionals I had consulted about my vision therapy, strabismus and side effects since commencing VT in January 2010 and I counted 14. Two developmental optometrists, three ophthalmologists, two neurologists, one neuro-ophthalmologist, two psychologists, one acupuncturist, one homeopath, one Ayurvedic doctor and a chiropractor specializing in cranial sacral therapy. Those cranial sacral treatments reduced my headaches, but the clinic itself was loud and hard for me to tolerate. When friends and family told me to get a second opinion, I laughed. I had already had many second opinions, more than ten of them. Most of the medical professionals had never even seen a case like mine. Being an enigma in medicine sucks. There was no better way to say it. I even tried a couple sessions with a hypnotherapist thinking that she could help me in case I had some medical block to find. Out of complete desperation, I contacted Ayurvedic medical centers in the south of India to see if they had experience with amblyopia, but I got the impression that they were just "spas" catering to Westerners. None of the doctors with whom I spoke had worked with patients such as myself. Ultimately, after many medical visits I, like Terzani, learned that the only person on whom I could rely was myself.

Ignorance is bliss

Accepting that only I could improve my life, I learned about how others overcame their 2D vision. I met a female surgeon at a reception and I asked her if she had ever worked with a doctor who could see with only one eye and who had no depth perception. I was curious if it was possible for someone to perform surgery and work with microscopes if they couldn't see depth.

To my great surprise, she told me that she saw with only one eye. She didn't have strabismus. Not only was she one of a minority of female surgeons with a child, she also was partially visually impaired. I was impressed.

A reader of my blog who was also strabismic wrote to me that his dream had always been to be a surgeon but he didn't think that he could do it because he lacked depth perception. I told him about the partially-blind surgeon whom I had met and that she had studied at Stanford Medical School, one of the most prestigious medical schools in the country. Even if we can't have precise depth perception like that of binocular people, it doesn't mean we can't live out our dreams, with a surgical knife in our hands or becoming a great salsa dancer!

Those of us who have never known what life is like in 3D may not even realize how we are limited in our abilities. We simply live and pursue our dreams just like anyone else.

When I told this to my friend Matt, he told me that when he explained to his father that I could only see in 2D, his father's automatic response was "How does she survive? How can she drive?"

"She doesn't know anything different than what she sees. She makes do and compensates in other ways."

When I lived in Argentina, one of my closest friends was a legally blind female lawyer, Cecilia. She traveled *on her own* in Europe and the US and always found people to help her.

People create all sorts of excuses for not doing things, and they are almost all based on fears or self-created complexes. If a blind woman could travel on her own and if a monocular person can perform surgeries, then there are no excuses!

Ignorance is bliss. Courage is gold.

More importantly though, speaking to the monocular surgeon made me feel empowered. Even if I didn't develop stereopsis, there was nothing "wrong" with the way I saw.

This reader's comment went right to the heart of my point in doing the best with what we have.

Commenter #14:

Hey there, Princess,

I just wanted to tell you that, yes, there is life after 3D. When I was 32, I had my first go at an auto-immune disorder called Eales Disease. At the time, I had 20/20 vision in both eyes. But in the...ahem... blink of an eye... I lost all the vision in my left eye. I was a trainer of hunter-jumper horses, a sport for which depth perception is critical because it is the rider who tells the horse when to leave the ground. Not being able to correctly "spot a distance" can have catastrophic results. Even 3D riders misjudge distances all the time, often with disastrous results. So I just assumed my riding career was over.

I then met a polo player from Argentina. One of the highest rated players in the world, he shocked me when he said a polo ball to the head had taken away the sight in one eye several years before. But with practice, he made a comeback. In fact, most people never knew he was gone. For years, he made an exceedingly brilliant and profitable career as a pro polo player.

I do remember being at a horse show in the early days after I lost my left eye sight. I came to a fence, misjudged the distance, and went flying, ass over tea kettle, as the quaint maxim goes. But I got back on. And with practice

I got better. I also got better at parking cars, stepping off curbs, filling a glass with liquid, and slicing fruit. In short, I learned to do all the things that anyone else can do.

And here's the kicker: about five years later, I lost the vision in my other eye. Completely. In the beat of a heart. Through some really good doctors and a lot of new research, I have been able to regain a fair amount of vision in my right eye. I now fluctuate between 2400 and 20/80–and I'm glad for every damn bit of it. I get injections in my eye every four weeks that help keep the condition under control and I also get Botox in the muscle of the left eye to keep it from rolling off to the side.

Many people, if not most, cannot tell that I have any vision issues, because I have pushed myself to adapt. Well, I don't have much choice–I have a great husband who has the worst bedside manner in the world and wouldn't stand for it if I whined. That bastard! Just kidding.

Anyway, we are rooting for you and know that you can make this struggle a force for good in the world. Already you are inspiring through the honesty, grace, dignity and wisdom with which you are handling this.

Yaaay, Princess!

Perseverance

Pushing to improve my vision and deal with handicaps involved stamina.

My optometrist shared an important lesson in perseverance one day when I walked into his office.

"I saw Sue Barry this weekend." He had attended the conference in Los Angeles for the College of Optometrists in Vision Development (COVD), where Sue Barry was a speaker and moderator.

"Her husband spoke at the conference as well and he told us about how he applied 14 times to be on a NASA Space Mission. After 14 times, he was accepted," Dr. K said with a smile.

"He never got his tenure at the university where he was teaching because he left to be an astronaut."

"But he realized his dream of being in space," I said.

The beauty of this story was that when Barry's husband told her about his space mission, she was fascinated by the visual aspect of it. When Barry attended a reception at NASA, she met Dr. Oliver Sacks whom she told about her inability to see in depth. Her husband encouraged her to write to Sacks when she was fascinated by the depth perception she had gained. After meeting Barry again, Dr. Sacks wrote "Stereo Sue," the article that changed my life. He also recommended that she find other people who had gone through a similar experience and write about it.

The moral of the story is to have resilience and to be persistent. If Barry's husband hadn't pursued his dream and continued to apply for the space missions despite his many rejections, Barry might have never contacted Dr. Sacks. If Dr. Sacks hadn't written the article "Stereo Sue," I'd still be in the dark about my vision.

Thank you to the Barrys for sticking to their dreams and to Dr. Sacks for writing and publishing!

Changing my thinking

I realized that I couldn't continue delaying what I wanted to do in my life because of the side effects of vision therapy.

I had several projects related to promoting foreign language learning and publishing that I decided would no longer be on the back burner and I would find ways to realize my dreams despite my mental and physical limitations.

Once I came to this realization, things around me changed. I quickly found two people with whom to collaborate on making some videos on YouTube to promote foreign language learning. The following week, a saxophonist who had been inviting me to his salsa concerts for months finally got me to go dance salsa. I had never danced so well in my life.

My vision also changed. I could see better even with my glasses off. Objects appeared to be sharper.

My energy came back. I didn't feel as lethargic. I also had fewer instances of confusing languages.

The ophthalmologist saw me after one year and told me that my eyes were straighter than before. While waiting for my appointment, I noticed the carpet in the waiting room and how the lighter colored patterns were raised above the darker ones. I got on my hands and knees to sit on the floor to closely examine the carpet to make sure that in fact the light colored patterns were not on the same level as the rest of the carpet. You know you are in binocular vision therapy when you have a newfound interest in waiting room carpets and you get into a crawling position to confirm your new visual perceptions!

Changing my inner perception of life and getting out of "being stuck" literally changed my vision.

Moving life to me

The cheiroscope exercise at UC Berkeley had always been the hardest for me. As I'd start tracing the image (a circle, a circle with a cross inside, a rectangle with a cross, etc.), I'd find that the reflection would change positions and I'd want to chase the new reflection and start my tracing at a new spot. Dr. Theis, the resident optometrist in binocular vision, said "Don't chase. Use your eyes to bring the image back to where you had it before."

I looked up and said, "Wow. That seems like good advice for my life outside of this office. Stop chasing and wait for things or make things to come to me." The doctor smiled.

Indeed, I often chased moving targets in life and got frustrated. I had no travel plans coming up and that was a good thing. I needed to stay put and get my eyes to be calm and work together. Chasing myself across time zones was not conducive to good binocular development.

Respite in words

"Siempre imaginé que el Paraíso sería algún tipo de biblioteca." ("I always imagined a library as a kind of paradise.")

- Jorge Luis Borges, Argentine writer

As I stopped chasing, I rediscovered what nurtured me intellectually and didn't irritate me.

In elementary school, my parents couldn't afford a babysitter so I was a latchkey kid. I walked myself to kindergarten when the school was across the street. At age seven we moved to another area, and I rode my bike to school, crossing major intersections. After school, since my parents couldn't afford after-school care, I would ride my bike to the nearest community center, right by the library in Almaden Valley in San Jose. Some days I had gymnastics, ballet or some other activity, and the other days I would go to the library, where I would read lots of books. On rainy days, the librarians would sometimes let my friends and me play hopscotch inside. The library became my babysitter and refuge; maybe that was one of the reasons I developed a strong vocabulary at a young age.

When I went to do vision therapy and my social activities had to cease, I went back to having the library as my "babysitter." After working in schools as a substitute teacher, I would go to the library and check out books. I would read the printed books and listen to the audio books when I went to the gym. I'd go on long walks in Mountain View and just listen to a book. The books became my entertainment and my babysitter. I was becoming who I was as a child, finding solace in books.

When I couldn't talk to people about what was happening, I wrote and didn't have to deal with people's interruptions. Hopefully, if a reader didn't understand something, they would just go back and read the previous paragraph and answer their question. I didn't have to deal with people rolling their eyes or looking away because they were bored with what I was saying. Also, I wouldn't get annoyed with what I thought were their stupid or repeated questions. It was in writing that I was able to communicate with others around the world who were amblyopes and/or in VT who also couldn't share about their vision with their friends and family. Ironically, as I was desiring to be able to see like others, I was becoming more aware of myself, fiercely protecting my honor via a literary sanctuary.

Wearing my Dr. Zhivago-esque coat, while admiring the snow-flakes in Armenia in February 2013, I wondered if the doctor/poet, Dr. Zhivago, played by Omar Sharif, would have enjoyed standing there with me to admire the snow, creating verses to describe the beauty of the falling flakes at night and in the day. Absent Boris Pasternak's literary protagonist by my side or his handsome Egyptian incarnation to accompany me in my wonderment, I had to become my own poet, even if I lacked the words to describe what I was seeing and feeling. I had to capture the images of the miraculous in my mind, storing them like a photo album until I could put into words the gorgeous new reality in front of me.

Developing a Sense of Self

I was talking to my friend David about how I felt that during my years of vision therapy, my life was deconstructed such that I had to pick up the pieces and decide what I wanted to be in my life. He said, "It's much like the Army. When people go through Basic Training, they're destroyed physically and mentally. They are pushed to the limits to do things they never thought they could do before."

I never thought I could do some of the vision things that I can do now. After I did them for the first time, I felt drained. David said, "Once they go through Basic Training and they develop experience, then they can specialize in what it is that they want to do, whether they want to be a radio technician, a linguist, etc."

I realized how doing vision therapy was kind of like Basic Training, but for my brain and eyes. Through my journey, I realized that I actually liked being an introvert. As my vision and side effects were becoming dominant factors in my life, I reverted to my introversion and silence to process the changes I saw and felt. Being an introvert and being guarded was much better for me than being an effusive extrovert. Reading and writing was not only a way to pass the time, but writing became my way to communicate. Vision therapy gave me an insight into my world that I would not have otherwise received.

When much of the world around me was unstable, either in duplicate, vibrating, moving or a combination of those and I couldn't find people who could support and understand me, the only person in whom I could confide and believe in was myself. Once I gave up on needing support or even acknowledgement from others, even though it was hard emotionally to distance myself from people who could never understand me, my road became easier. I relied only on myself. I was done with excusing and explaining myself.

Instead of feeling lonely when surrounded by people who couldn't or wouldn't understand or respect me, I found happiness in being alone most of the time and only sharing my world with the few who did "get" me. I had to rely on myself to be my own healer, counselor, cheerleader, best friend and Dr. Zhivago.

Feeling lonely, unappreciated and misunderstood is miserable.

Being happy alone is a joyous and liberating experience.

– CHAPTER SIX –

Advice

In my years of doing VT, I've learned many lessons about what to do and what not to do. Since many of the struggles adult VT patients have are regarding how to deal with people in their lives who don't have the condition, I have written advice for both the patient and those supporting the patient based on my experiences and those of others. At risk of repeating some of the information in previous chapters, I assembled all of tips in this section for easy reference.

The three most important things to remember when considering surgery and vision therapy are:

1) **Find an experienced optometrist trained in binocular vision therapy.**

2) **Find an ophthalmologist with a background in binocular vision issues.**

3) **Locate an optician who has experience with asymmetric eyes.**

The following sections have advice on buying prism glasses, VT and Dos and Don'ts.

On Purchasing Prism Eye Glasses

Be careful when getting prism glasses and ask the optician if he/she has experience with prism glasses. Ask your doctor which lens dispensary he/she recommends and trusts for filling prism prescriptions.

IMPORTANT!!!

In their practice, opticians use a tool called a pupillometer which measures pupillary distance (PD) in order to center the lenses on the patient's visual axis. Make sure the optician does not make their own pupillometer measurement of your eyes. The optician's PD measurement may not be the same as that of the developmental optometrist. The difference in the PD measurement can have disastrous effects on your prescription.

If "homicide by optician error" exists in the legal code, it almost happened to me.

I am not exaggerating when I say that what I experienced could have been fatal.

After two and a half LONG years in VT, I finally got a prescription for prism glasses in mid-May, 2012. I went to a popular eyeglasses chain near my home to fill the prescription and after a long delay, I received a pair that almost caused me to crash my car because the pupillary distance was incorrectly calculated by the optician.

Effect: I had to drive with one eye closed because my left field of vision moved faster than my right field. The divider lanes on the left doubled at a 20 degree angle into my lane, causing me to get confused as to where my lane was. At night, the extra divider

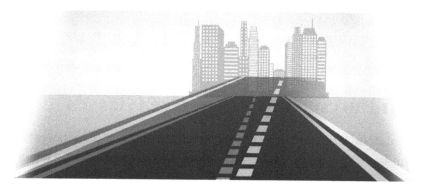

The left lane doubled at a 20° angle and was elevated.

lane was not only at a 20 degree angle but it was sometimes elevated above ground. Driving with one eye closed is difficult.

I couldn't look down when descending a staircase because the end of the step would also double at a 20 degree angle, making it hard for me to see where the end of each step was. Other lines, whether they were on sidewalks or my kitchen floor, would double or be distorted.

Problem: After trying another pair of glasses which were also wrong, the optometrist in the chain store compared my developmental optometrist's original prescription with what had been entered into the computer.

My doctor had originally prescribed a PD of 60mm. The optician, following "standard operating procedure," had measured my PD for each eye with a pupillometer, and came to a total PD of 56mm. She overrode my doctor's PD calculation and entered her PD measurement into the computer prescription. The missing 4mm in the PD altered the horizontal prism in the glasses and made my life extremely difficult.

Those 4mm could have caused a car accident because of my distorted vision.

Solution:

Blood boiling, I called the chain's corporate headquarters to rectify this matter. After I put up quite a fight, including threatening them with a medical malpractice lawsuit, they reimbursed me for my various doctor's office visits because of the incorrect glasses and paid me for damages as I had lost two months of my VT. Unfortunately, the chain didn't take me seriously until I told them that I had discussed the issue with an attorney.

If something similar happens to you and the optician and optician's supervisor don't treat you with respect and reimburse you for your visits, you can tell them that you will report their mistake to the Medical Board, the state agency which issues licenses for opticians and optical dispensaries. The words "medical malpractice lawsuit" tend to make people return your phone calls.

Impact on strabismics and amblyopes:

The chain eyeglasses store said they informed their optician trainers about the issue. (Their legal department was also aware, as they handled my case.) But I will never find out if the opticians will indeed ever get any training on how to measure the PD for strabismics and amblyopes. An estimated 3% of the population has amblyopia and/or strabismus. Since not everyone in the general population requires corrective lenses, but almost all strabismics and amblyopes do, more than 3% of any optical store's potential clients have misaligned eyes and could be at risk of causing accidents if wearing glasses that are incorrectly measured by opticians. I wonder about all the other opticians in the country. Could they all be incorrectly measuring PD and dispensing harmful glasses?

On supporting people with binocular vision issues

If you are supporting someone with binocular vision issues, please read the following tips to learn about what to do and not to do. It is wonderful that you want to know what life is like for your friend or relative doing VT. Getting support from loved ones is fundamental. Your support and mindfulness could make your friend's life much easier. I use the words "friend" or "patient" to refer to VT patients and those with binocular vision problems.

I know that people in my life were frustrated because they didn't know what to do to help me, and they were confused by my negative reactions to their pep talks and actions. I wrote this section of the book to prevent others from having the same problems I had.

1. **Sometimes what you may earnestly be doing to help a VT patient may unintentionally frustrate them and you may not understand why.**

It's important for you to **not** think about how **you** would like to be treated if you were a VT patient. Instead, ask how **your friend/spouse/loved one/colleague** how **they** prefer to be treated.

Don't assume what could help. Ask.

You may think that driving your friend to and from sessions is the best way to help them. Please consider that if you are prone to talking a lot or listening to the radio in the car, the noise may disturb them. It is common for people to be tired after VT sessions, have a headache, feel disoriented, be nauseated, and/or have other side effects. A chatty friend may make the VT patient uncomfortable. It's hard to tell someone who is doing you a favor to be quiet, but your silence may be exactly what your friend needs. Before asking about all the details about the VT session, their work day, love/relationship gossip, or whatever else, ask if they want to talk, listen to music or just be silent. If you know that you have trouble being silent for a long time, do not volunteer to drive a friend who requires exactly that, otherwise your friend may not only feel uncomfortable with too much talking, but also guilty for having made you drive in silence, when all you wanted to do was chat.

The boyfriend of one female VT patient thought he was assuaging her frustration by saying, "We'll get through this together." But she was the one who had to do the VT exercises and resented his pep talk.

Be mindful of your friend's personality type. If they are the type of person who needs to externalize their thoughts and brainstorm, then accept that this is the way they are processing their visual changes. If your friend needs to ponder before speaking, don't press them for answers, give them space. Know their boundaries.

2. **Relating to people with binocular vision problems.**

It's common for people to try to relate another person's life to their own life experience. **Do not** attempt to reframe your amblyopic friend's stories into your life. Unless you have a hidden disability or have had an intense neurological intervention or brain trauma, you will most likely not be able to fit your struggles to theirs.

Although something as innocuous as, "When I was 10 and broke my right arm, I had to write my class assignments with my left hand and that was really hard because I am right handed," may seem like a way of relating, it is not. Even though you may be right handed, you always used your left hand for other activities. It's not as though the first time you had to use your left hand was at the age of 10 after the accident. If someone is going through VT and has never used one of their eyes, they are starting from zero in terms of using their eye muscles and their brains. They are waking up dormant binocular brain cells.

Making comparisons to your own life experience may belittle what your friend is telling you and may make them feel like you don't understand. When someone with binocular vision problems feels misunderstood, they may feel even more isolated and less inclined to share their experience. If your friend is describing something that is extremely painful emotionally, consider just listening and asking how you can be of assistance.

3. If you're not listening, be upfront.

If you're not in a state of mind to listen attentively and pay attention to your friend when they are telling you about their experience, don't fake it. There's no use pretending to listen when you are not. It's better to be upfront about your limitation than for your friend to cry out their heart to you for two hours and then find out that you neither recall a word they said nor understand them. If you repeatedly ask the same questions and don't remember the answers, your friend may get aggravated and may decide to completely shut off and not share with you again. You may not understand why they are angry at you for not listening and remembering. If you know you have a bad memory or have trouble understanding medical details and won't be able to retain most of what the person is saying, be upfront. Adult VT patients may be working through childhood trauma about being teased for their divergent eyes, eye patches, thick glasses or memories from surgery. If these topics are too heavy for you, be honest.

4. Remember that there are very few doctors trained in binocular vision therapy.

If you know a VT patient who has to take time off of work, sleep over at a friend's place, and travel far away for doctor's appointments, asking why they don't just go to the optometrist down the street from their house may seem like an innocent and obvious question, but it could be annoying for them to hear.

VT patients have enough trouble driving and some of them may not even drive at all. If they are going to a doctor two hours away, they have most likely already researched their local optometrists to determine who can help them. They know there are optometrists in their city. The thing that you may not know is that none of those optometrists are trained in VT. Some patients fly across the country or from other countries to visit trained optometrists who specialize in binocular vision.

People often asked me these types of questions: "Why don't you go to Stanford Medical School? It's so much closer to your house." "What about X hospital, X clinic, etc.?" No matter how many times I told them that Stanford didn't have an Optometry School or that X hospital didn't have vision therapy facilities, I would still get the same questions and they would make my blood boil. If the choice of a closer eye doctor were so easy, I would have thought of those "logical" options long ago.

If you do want to know why your friend/relative has selected a doctor far away, it is best to just ask, "Why did you choose this doctor?" instead of framing the question as a judgment on the patient.

If you want to help find a closer option, look for optometrists trained in binocular vision therapy on www.covd.org.

5. **Accompanying the patient to VT sessions.**

If you're a parent of a young child, the doctor may require your presence in sessions to make sure your child behaves and for you to provide support. Your child may get easily frustrated by the exercises and may need your assurance. Ask the doctor what you need to do to prepare your child before sessions and support them during therapy.

(If you know you have a loud child, please do your best to keep him or her quiet as there could be other patients in the office working hard who could be bothered by your child's outbursts.)

If the VT patient is an adult, ask if the patient wants you to be there with him or her while he/she is doing the exercises.

Some adults may appreciate the support. However, for an adult VT patient, having their friend watch them struggle to draw a triangle using a cheiroscope or merge two objects projected on the screen while wearing funny prism glasses may be embarrassing and put pressure on the patient to "perform." Even if you say nothing and are just sitting there playing on your smartphone or are reading a book, your presence may be a distraction.

6. **Ask what activities the patient can do before you think of what would work for them.**

   Ask open-ended questions to elicit an answer. Your friend may actually be confused about what he/she is able to do. Probe to help your friend figure out which activities are both pleasant and possible.

   If the patient gets nauseated, don't plan outings to go dancing or to amusement parks with Ferris wheels and roller coasters on the days the patient has VT sessions.

   Noise sensitivity is a common side effect of vision therapy. If the patient says that they can't go to a party because it will be too noisy, **don't try** to cajole them into attending. You will make them feel even worse and guilty for not going.

   Recognizing their limitations and voicing that you remember that they can't do X, Y, or Z shows the patient that you are listening and that you care. Asking what they want to do is a good way to show that you want them to feel comfortable and that you want to find ways to spend time together.

7. **Plan appropriate outings.**

   One man, trying to court me, told me he'd teach me to play tennis, as he was a tennis pro. I didn't want to explain my vision to him, but I was adamant (in a nice way) that I wasn't interested in his tennis lessons. People with binocular vision problems often have hand-eye coordination problems. Add that to our limited depth perception, and you'll see that hitting a ball with a tennis racket can be a frustrating and futile endeavor when the brain can't figure out how far away the ball is, causing the player to constantly hit the air instead of the tennis ball. Squash and ping pong can also be challenging. Golf and billiards (pool) require depth perception to shoot the balls correctly. Hiking or walking on unstable ground or on unflat surfaces can be challenging, as the VT patient may have trouble figuring out where it is safe to step. Avoid inviting VT patients to these activities unless you already know that they enjoy them.

Daytime activities are the best so the VT patient doesn't have to worry about binocular vision issues that are worse at night. A daytime walk or hike on the beach or a paved/smooth road is a good option. Sports like cycling, jogging, or swimming are preferable because they don't require hand-eye coordination. If your friend is having noise tolerance issues, pick locations (restaurants, cafés, bars and museums) during off-peak hours when it is less likely to be noisy. Concerts, (2D) movies, or theatrical performances could also be good options as long as they are not too loud.

8. Offer to drive to social events.

If you know that driving and parking, especially at night, are difficult for your VT friend, then offer to drive or take public transportation together. Especially if your friend is an independent person, they may not feel comfortable asking for rides. If you offer, it might make them feel more open to going out.

9. Preface your invitations.

Let's say your friend doing VT hasn't been able do a certain activity (like dancing, be in a loud bar or focus on a sporting event as a spectator) but may be able to do it every once in a while when their side effects are mild. Preface your invitation by saying something like, "I know your vision makes it difficult to do _____ (activity), but sometimes you are able; do you think you might be up for going to _____ with our friends this weekend?" This way, you are not excluding your friend and you are showing that you remember their limitations. Otherwise, if you just invite them thinking that you are being inclusive, they could possibly get hurt that you forgot that they can't do _____ activity.

10. Be mindful of what you say and write in public.

To avoid humiliating yourself and your friend, ask your friend what kinds of subjects they are sensitive about, and whether it's okay to mention certain medical information in public.

Some people with binocular vision issues can see the 3D effects in 3D movies. I can't. Getting an email invitation sent to a group of people about seeing a 3D movie was like rock salt on a deep wound. Having to respond to everyone on the group email that I couldn't go to the movie because I couldn't see in 3D was deeply mortifying. Although I didn't have to admit why I couldn't go to the 3D movie, I did it so that the others on the email thread, who already knew I couldn't see in 3D, wouldn't make the same mistake by inviting me to such an event in the future. Think before publically inviting your friend to activities and sports that are beyond their reach.

If you are at a group event and you want to introduce your friend to someone else to discuss their issues, ask your friend in private if he/she wants to talk about their medical situation with others. Just because your friend tells you information, it doesn't mean that they want to share it with strangers.

Once, I was in the middle back seat of the car when a friend tried to get me to talk about my eye issues to the driver of the vehicle, a lady I had just met that day. Not only was I not inclined to divulge my medical history to an almost-stranger but I was physically stuck in the middle back seat with no place to go. At least at a party, I could go and talk to other people or leave, but in the car, I was not just in a physically uncomfortable position, but also in a socially awkward one. I had to say "no" twice for my friend to get the message that I wasn't going to talk about VT.

Pause before you open your mouth or press "send" in an email, especially an email sent to a group of people when the topic deals with a person's disability or an activity your friend can't do.

11. **Just because you can't see a hidden disability doesn't mean it's not real.**

a. An invisible challenge is still a challenge.

b. Just because a person doesn't LOOK like they're struggling in a certain area doesn't mean that they aren't.

Telling a friend with binocular vision issues that you forgot that they can't do X activity due to their vision issues because it's hard for you to fathom that they are limited is not an excuse for not remembering and respecting their situation. You may think it's OK to say to them that they are so successful in other areas of their life and you admire them for their abilities. This may sound like a way of praising your friend or cheering them up, but it can come across as an excuse for being irresponsible.

If somebody has confided to you that they have trouble walking down stairs, parallel parking, playing tennis or performing some other activity due to their vision issues, they have trusted you with this information which they most likely do not make public. (Some people are very open about their limitations and may not have problems with others knowing about their disability.) It can be embarrassing for an adult to admit how hard it is for them to drive or walk down stairs. Make a concerted effort to remember these things. Just because they live on the 4th floor of an elevator-less building, read voraciously, drive a car, and appear to look just fine doesn't mean that those activities are super easy for them. Be patient if they walk slowly and deliberately down the stairs.

A close family member of mine told me she thought I was a hypochondriac because I appeared fine. I had to enlist the help of my two strabismic aunts who don't drive on highways or at night. They sat down with the naysayer and explained how incredibly difficult their day-to-day lives were in terms of their limited depth perception in order for the naysayer to take me seriously.

12. Are you sure you can't see in 3D?

People have asked me this question on many occasions because they can't believe that I can function and be able to travel as much as I do and even drive if I am monocular.

"Who told you that you can't see in 3D?" the inquiring mind asked.

"My eye doctor, of course," I replied.

If your friend tells you that he has trouble driving because he can't see in depth, believe him even if his eyes are straight.

Testing someone's 3D vision at home with 3D lenses and a 3D video on YouTube or on TV can potentially be humiliating to a VT patient. Unless the patient offers to prove that they can't see the *Avatar* movie on your 3D TV in 3D, please don't make them testify. Some people with normal binocular vision have trouble with 3D movies.

13. "Your eyes look fine to me. Why are you doing this therapy?"

Your friend whose eyes look straight (either because they've been surgically straightened or have an almost imperceptible asymmetry) is not doing VT to be in an ocular beauty pageant. Those who have asymmetric eyes may be doing the therapy to straighten their eyes to look "normal." Some amblyopes don't have asymmetry but one eye could be far-sighted and the other near-sighted. These types of patients pursue VT to develop depth perception. The rest of the patients who do have asymmetric eyes are doing the therapy to straighten their eyes, to see better and/or make their life easier. I've had people try to make me feel better by telling me how much they like my eyes. Their words had an opposite effect; they showed me that they didn't understand my aim for doing the therapy. I wanted to see in depth, not parade around my eyes! Besides, those who do vision therapy and have to wear prism glasses in order for their eyes to work together are not going to be wearing their contact lenses anymore because contacts don't have prisms. If you want more time staring into your amblyopic lover's naked eyes, think again! Most likely the amblyope will be spectacled so he/she can see you in more depth.

Accept your friend's desire and commitment to VT as part of their own journey.

14. Be careful with your advice.

Unless you are a medical professional in the field of optometry, ophthalmology or neurology, or you have your own binocular issues, you most likely do not have the medical basis to give informed advice. Even other amblyopes may not always give the right advice because there are lots of differences among patients and what works for one patient may not work for another.

Before sharing unsolicited medical recommendations, consider the impact of your words.

Most medical eye doctors (ophthalmologists) deal with the pathology of the eyes and do not support optometric vision therapy which is carried out by optometrists. Optometrists focus on the function of the eyes. Your grandmother's cataracts specialist is most likely not a specialist in strabismus or amblyopia and is not trained to judge the VT patient's situation. You will only make matters worse by recommending doctors who are not capable of helping a VT patient.

Perhaps you have seen some promotions for LASIK surgery or you know of a new doctor offering discounts for laser eye surgery and perhaps you think that this quick and easy surgery will help your friend enjoy a spectacle-less life. You are wrong. Before waxing poetic about how wonderful it is to live without glasses or contacts and waking up in the morning and seeing everything clearly and in its place, bear in mind that a VT patient is working on both their brain **and** their eyes. No laser surgery to date can wake up dormant binocular brain cells and change the way the brain takes in the images from two asymmetric eyes.

15. **Try your friend's VT exercises.**

One year, at Thanksgiving, I brought my **Bernell Mirror Stereoscope (Batwing)** and **tranaglyphs** with red-green glasses to show my relatives my divergence and convergence exercises. I didn't expect to be the entertainment of the evening, but I was touched by the one person, my cousin's wife Olga, who actually took an interest in the exercises and asked how they worked. The other adults tried the exercises, said their eyes felt strained or they were getting a headache, and left.

Oddly enough, I was at a memorial service after a family funeral and some relatives asked me about my VT. They asked to try my exercises with the red-green glasses and the vectograms. To my surprise, they had fun figuring out how it all worked. I don't suggest bringing along VT homework to funerals as a regular practice!

If you make a sincere effort to do the exercises with your friend you might see in double and feel the eye strain, fatigue and headaches, which may make you better able to empathize with your friend's predicament.

This doesn't mean you have to hurt or sacrifice yourself! You are stepping into your friend's world and that effort will be appreciated.

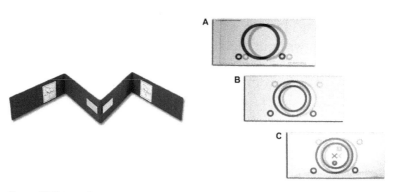

Bernell Mirror. Stereoscope (Batwing) and tranaglyphs.
Images credit: ©Bernell Corporation

16. **"My friend is also an amblyope and doesn't care about seeing in 3D so why is it such a big deal to you?"**

If someone has made the commitment to do VT, rest assured that it was not a capricious decision, especially if the patient is an adult who has to pay for the sessions from their own funds.

An adult who decides to do VT wants to improve their vision and life. Depth perception helps one perform activities as simple as walking down the stairs and pouring water from a pitcher into a glass, to harder tasks like merging in traffic.

I have two strabismic aunts who don't care about seeing in 3D. However, they support my doing VT to learn to see with both eyes. They use only one eye and if something happens to their good eye, they will be in major trouble as they will be practically blind with their bad eye.

My aunts are homebodies. I am not. I am extremely active and am often traveling. I want to see the world. Our decisions about our vision are based on our priorities and aspirations. I don't fault my aunts for not doing VT. Their disinterest in VT and depth perception has had no sway in my commitment to improving my vision, nor should it.

Not every amblyope feels their life to be severely impacted by amblyopia, or they've learned to overcome the obstacles by some other means.

Just because you know someone who is fine with their 2D world doesn't mean that another person's pursuit of 3D vision is not a valid choice and not one worth supporting. Trying to sway a VT patient away from their dream with reasoning based on someone else's life and priorities is not supportive.

Your amblyopic aunt may see more or less depth than your friend who is doing VT. Remember that the level of depth perception varies from one amblyope to another.

17. **If you're a fixer, come to terms, right now, with the fact that binocular vision issues are not a medical condition you can fix.**

I am a practical person, the daughter of two engineers. I grew up in Silicon Valley, the land where visionaries think they can solve many of the world's problems with an app, software or some digital device. Not all problems are so easily solvable.

Steve Jobs, the co-founder of Apple Computers, died of pancreatic cancer. If he could have come up with a gadget to cure pancreatic cancer, I would wager that he would have poured his fortunes into the technology.

Unfortunately, there's no easy solution yet for strabismus. Researchers and technology professionals are working on 3D video games for improving depth perception, but, although promising for some people, that technology has not been completely proven as sufficient. Nor is it totally safe for VT patients to play 3D video games without the supervision of a trained optometrist. It is possible to develop diplopia by doing video games when not directed by an experienced doctor. VT equipment for home use can be bought only with an optometrist's prescription.

If you're reading this book, it's because you want to help someone with binocular vision problems or because a VT patient asked you to read this section of the book. If you're the type of person who likes to fix problems, join the club! I am a problem solver as well and I've been wrapping my head around this issue for over five years. Despite researchers looking for possible ways to help those of us with unaligned eyes see in stereo, there are no clear-cut solutions which work for everybody. Each amblyope has a unique set of circumstances. Some are far-sighted, others near-sighted.

Others have eye problems like astigmatism which affect their vision therapy.

If you want to learn more about the mechanics of vision therapy, I encourage you to read Dr. Sue Barry's book, *Fixing My Gaze*. If you truly want to delve into the details of past and current research on the condition, you can look up medical research articles online.

The best thing you can do is be a good listener for the VT patient in your life.

18. **Although you may not be able to "do" much to help, it's who you are being that will make a difference.**

Being supportive may mean doing nothing more than allowing the VT patient the space to discover a new world. You don't have to hold their hand, understand the neuro-ophthalmological details of how their brain is changing, ask them about all of their exercises, or even try on their weird-looking prism glasses. If you do sport the glasses, be ready to laugh at your reflection in the mirror.

A VT patient is likely to encounter many changes in their life. I only know one who got away without fatigue, headaches, nausea or other side effects, but the majority of us have major side effects.

No matter if your friend is suffering from double vision or other side effects, their changing vision does impact their life. Be patient with them if you're in the park and they spend a lot of time staring at trees. Many of us in VT admire tree branches. Maybe the VT patient needs to admire trees and other plant life in silence. Let them do just that and don't rush them. Allowing them to take in their newly forming world without your judgment or haste may be the best show of support you can give. Imagine a baby coming into the world and playing with the toys dangling from the crib or a young child delighting in riding a school bus for the first time. The baby's eyes dance as the toys move around. A few times when I was with people and I wanted some time alone to stare at snowflakes or flies, I felt like I was inconveniencing them. One of them couldn't stop talking when I told him to give me a few minutes to look at white flies in the park. Ask if it's better to be quiet.

What a VT patient needs more than anything is feeling supported. While you may not be able to finance the therapy sessions, you can be there to let them feel comfortable taking in their new world. What you may see as mundane or even annoying, like looking at dew on flower petals, could be a treasure chest of new visual experiences for a VT patient. If the VT patient can't find the words to describe what they see, that's fine. I often found myself, a multilingual writer, at a loss for words in any language to describe what I was seeing. Sometimes I didn't even know why I was staring at things like orange peels or toilet paper. Don't expect explanations.

19. Respect their confidence in you.

It is not uncommon for strabismic and amblyopic people to not want to talk about their vision issues. Especially for those of us who have had our eyes surgically straightened, we may prefer people not know of our issue. Therefore, if someone does open up to you about their eyes and limitations in life, take it as a sign that they trust you and feel comfortable enough to share this deeply personal information. It is possible that you may be one of very few people who know their secret. Being a person of confidence carries a responsibility or weight. Granted, you may not be keen on being this person of confidence. Even if the VT patient's newfound ability to appreciate snow or flying dust sounds juvenile, minor, or even stupid to you, take the time to feel what it is like for them to tell you about this "trivial" thing which is so important to them. They might even feel embarrassed to reveal that they spent 30 minutes in the bathroom staring at mildew, admiring the texture of their toilet paper or looking at how the drops of water on their shower curtain stood out against the color of the curtain. What they are telling you may not be easy for them to admit. They are being extremely vulnerable and if this is too much for you to handle, be honest.

20. Don't assume our lives are boring because we can't see in 3D.

On more than one occasion, people have told me that if they could only see in 2D, life would be boring and lifeless. Before the advent of 3D movies and TV, you didn't avoid television and the cinema because the images were only in 2D. Though some people who don't see in 3D may have boring lives, the monotony of their lives is not a result of their vision, it's because of other factors and personal choices.

Gordon Brown was Prime Minister of the UK from 2007-2010 and had governed the country during the financial crisis of 2008. He can only see in 2D because he's blind in one eye. (He's not strabismic.) Although I've never met the man, I can assure you that when he was Prime Minister, life was anything **but** boring. Now with his roles at the World Economic Forum and as the United Nations Special Envoy on Global Education, his world is probably complicated and fascinating. There are highly successful people who have hidden disabilities. Charles Schwab, the head of the investment company in his name, is dyslexic, as is the founder of Ikea. Beethoven composed Symphony No. 9 when he was almost deaf.

Unless someone who was born with 3D vision had an accident which left them without vision in one eye, and can vividly recall life before 2D, those of us with 2D vision know no other way of seeing. It is probably more difficult for us to imagine how you see with two eyes than for you to envision how we see the world. Some of you can close one eye and you'll see in 2D, while other people can close one eye and still see in 3D because their brains fill in the missing information.

21. "If driving is so hard for you, why don't you move to a metropolitan area and use public transportation?"

It's not that easy. Do you think that everyone who has amblyopia who does not already reside in a city is going to drop everything in their life to move to the nearest metropolis with good public transportation? People have work, family and personal reasons to live where they are. Not everyone likes urban living, congestion and bad air pollution. Many of us have noise sensitivities and would have trouble dealing with the constant noise in a big city.

22. Don't be a backseat driver

You may feel like you are on high alert now every time you are the passenger in your amblyopic's friend's car since you have read how hard it is to merge and park. If you truly feel uncomfortable, ask your friend if they need your directions to help them merge and park. If they don't want the directions and you don't feel comfortable, then just don't go in their vehicle. Getting turn-by-turn backseat directions may be more of a nuisance than a service. If you know they have trouble parking, offer to park their car and/or get their car out of tight parking spots for them.

23. If you can't understand what they describe, ask them to draw it

If your friend's explanations of double vision, vibrating images and displaced images don't make sense to you, ask them to draw it for you. When I showed people the Dalí painting I described in the introduction to this book, some said, "Oh, this is what you mean by double vision" because none of my previous descriptions made any sense to them. Your friend may not be a painting maestro, but they can at least draw stick figure drawings for you to get an idea of what they are seeing. If your friend knows how to manipulate photos on the computer, then they may be able to use a photo editing program to alter photos to show double images or other visual aberrations. Don't ask them to just take photos of what they see because photos are 2D and reflect what the camera lenses see, not what your friend's brain and eyes are showing them.

On doing VT (for the patient)

1. **Be careful about those with whom you share your VT stories.**

   At the same time that I encourage people to be vocal about what it is like being monocular, I caution them to first honor themselves and not put themselves in uncomfortable situations.

   For most people who see in 3D, our explanations of life in flatland fall on deaf ears.

   I have few regrets in life. One of them is speaking with as many people as I did about vision therapy.

   The sad truth is that talking to people about a world they can't imagine is a colossal waste of time. This may leave you feeling depleted and even more alienated than before. Feeling isolated has been the most difficult part of being in VT and about explaining binocular vision issues.

   Don't burden your friends with the details of clown vectograms, Brock string exercises and prisms, unless you know that they will do their best to understand you.

Choose people whom you think would be more supportive. People who have had to make major life changes, voluntarily or involuntarily, and have succeeded, are much better conversation candidates.

It is hard to leave people out, but if you know that they have neither the capacity to listen nor the life experience or intelligence to process what you are saying and at least try to imagine your predicament, it is better to save these heavy conversations for those people who do have the ability to listen. They may not comprehend, but at least you know they will listen, remember and respect you.

Unfortunately, and I say this with deep sorrow, you may have to cut off a major part of yourself from the people around you. What is worse is that they may be the closest to you (your family and best friends).

Friends and family may confide in you about profound topics like their careers, relationships, spiritual battles and impending divorces or more everyday topics like which washing machine to buy, and you can understand what they are discussing. However, your stories about rewiring your brain and seeing the walls vibrate are galaxies beyond their ability or desire to comprehend or empathize. This creates an unequal relationship where you may feel cheated and isolated. Perhaps, over time, you'll find ways to convey your thoughts and feelings in such a way that others will 'get' you.

Search for others who have your condition. Go to www. sovoto.com and join the Adults Strabismics Forum. Write to VT bloggers. Find people in your area with whom you can meet. When I joined a research lab for amblyopes as a research subject, I was overjoyed to meet adults with whom I could share experiences, one of whom became a carpool partner and friend. The pressure to communicate about my changing world with my friends and family diminished because I had a cohort which shared my experience in the lab, and I didn't have to struggle to explain to them what I saw and felt. It took me four and a half years in VT to find this community. Before that I had met people on the Internet with my condition and I had people to write to but I didn't have a physical meeting place where I'd always find someone like me. If you can't find others in your geographical area, make an effort to speak to people by Skype or phone. Having this support is of utmost importance. When no one in your immediate circle of friends and family can understand you, it is healthy to at least have Internet acquaintances who don't think you are loony when you say you see two moons.

2. **Don't explain, don't complain.**

VT hasn't just changed what and how I see, it has also made me take my side effects into account when making choices about my career, relationships, travel and social life. Often times, explaining my rationale for my decisions confuses people and they prefer to debate me rather than understand my predicament.

One of my strabismic aunts told me "Don't explain. Don't complain," meaning don't bother explaining your life or else you'll end up complaining that people don't get it. For those people I know who cannot even fathom what I am going through, I don't explain why I can't go to certain events or perform certain activities. There's no use in making up lies. However, if you have to keep using the same excuse that you're sick, have a headache or are tired, it is easier than burning yourself out with explanations. Or don't give an excuse at all.

3. **Don't expect people to understand. Seek support and love, not understanding. The most you can get is respect and you're lucky if you get even that.**

My father said, "don't expect people to understand. It's useless. Few people have the empathy to step into someone else's shoes and experience the world as they do."

Doing VT as an adult is already an experience that makes you feel alone, especially when you're the only adult in the doctor's office and the kids are jumping on the trampoline that your optometrist doesn't let you jump on because you are too tall and you could hit your head on the ceiling.

If an individual keeps bugging you with the same questions and comments and advice, ask them to respect that you don't want to discuss your medical situation with them anymore. The book, *Living with a Hidden Disability*, has tips on tactful ways to get people to stop bothering you and giving you unsolicited advice.

The most we can ask for is for people to respect our limitations. After struggling for many years to get a close family member to stop asking me to drive her long distances at night, I have to admit that getting a "simple" recognition of my limitations is an arduous task.

4. **If someone really wants to understand the neuro-ophthalmology behind VT, have them read Sue Barry's *Fixing My Gaze*, listen to her NPR interview and watch her TED talk about her journey.**

Dr. Barry is both a neurobiologist and a strabismic success story. She explains the neurobiology behind VT and gives her own examples of how she gained stereopsis. Having your loved ones read her book may take the load off of you.

5. Be prepared for your life to change dramatically, including in ways you cannot predict.

In 2010 when I started VT I had the crazy idea that I was both going to gain 3D vision and become a great salsa dancer. As I found out by getting dizzy and falling in salsa clubs, those two activities were contra-indicated.

If you are a party person, you may become super sensitive to noise and smells after doing VT sessions and your party days may be limited or over.

Don't over-schedule yourself on a day with a VT session. One thirty-minute VT session can give you a massive headache for the rest of the day. You may wake up the next day with a headache. Doing nothing after a VT session or just going for a walk is a good idea. Slow down.

If you have plans after a VT session, make sure those with whom you made plans know that you may have to cancel. You don't have to go into detail about VT when explaining why you may have to reschedule. Just telling your friends that you will have a medical procedure and that you may not feel well afterwards should be enough information.

After starting VT, I found myself often falling asleep during movies. I'd see the characters on screen in double and my brain would get so tired of shutting off the double image that my brain just made me sleep even if I wasn't tired.

Some VT patients don't experience sudden sleepiness like I did, but be prepared for major disruptions to your life, including nausea, headaches, fatigue, noise sensitivity, or double vision that make reading very difficult. You may even experience reduced tolerance of annoyances or speech problems.

If you have a demanding job and busy family life, the side effects of VT could dramatically affect your ability to function at work and at home. Be realistic. If you are unable to allow yourself to sleep 10-12 hours a day to recover from rewiring your brain, you may suffer major fatigue throughout the day, impeding your work, studies, and domestic responsibilities. You may have to temporarily cease certain activities to allow yourself the recovery time your brain needs to assimilate changes.

6. Sleep!

Your performance will be much worse if you don't get enough sleep. Your brain needs to be rested and alert to do VT because you are waking up parts of your brain which have been dormant most or all of your life. If you feel sleepy, so does your brain. VT is expensive. Make sure to maximize your VT sessions by being energetic.

7. Be prepared with food and caffeine.

Vision therapy is super tiring for the brain. It's like mental gymnastics.

A VT session is making you change the way your brain has always worked. Don't pack your day with activities and think you can go to VT after work and then go grocery shopping, do errands, see friends, take a class, etc. You may be absolutely exhausted or mentally confused after your session, so much so that you may need to walk to the nearest cafe and get a coffee or other caffeinated or sweet drink to keep you functional. I sometimes needed coffee or tea before, during or after a session. I saw an elderly lady drink Red Bull to stay alert in VT. Bring a thermos, mug, cup or other receptacle with the beverage you need to stay alert.

DO NOT drink alcohol before, during or after VT or else your brain will not be at its best.

If you need snacks to keep you going, bring them in small and easy-to-reach bags or containers.

8. **If you're in a VT office with kids and are sensitive to noise, bring noise cancellation headphones or ear plugs.**

    Adults doing VT have an extra difficult task of focusing. Noise from kids can make VT all the more strenuous.

    Schedule your VT when there are no children in the office. This can be difficult if you prefer to come in at the end of the day after work, when kids come in after school. Mornings are usually quieter but if you have to go to work after VT, you may be drained and unable to concentrate. Some VT offices offer Saturday appointments.

9. **Do your VT exercises at home with kids.**

    Explaining my VT exercises to adults seemed silly because most adults didn't understand what I was doing. But my niece and nephew loved playing with my prisms and prism glasses and seeing people in double. They would watch me do my exercises and note down my scores. They became my coaches, or as they preferred to be called, my "butt kickers" because they kicked my butt (figuratively) to work harder and beat my previous scores.

    When you are doing VT as an adult, you can revert to being a child because many of the exercises feature characters from children's stories, like Humpty Dumpty. Think of yourself as a child who is learning to see. Doing the exercises with kids takes away the embarrassment and tedium.

10. **Allow yourself to be a child.**

    Part of the beauty of VT is experiencing life with (literally) new eyes, like a child. Who else will stare at the ridges in toilet paper or marvel at the rain drops on a flower? When small things that nobody else cares about rock your world, let yourself be like a child exploring a new world. Maybe you have to spend your lunch break alone in a park looking at tree branches. If being a kid is not socially acceptable or you feel awkward telling people around you how excited you are to see white flies you have never seen before, reserve time to be alone.

11. **Have compassion for those in your life who are trying to be of support to you but don't know how to help you.**

There are people who will sincerely try to do what they can to help you, but what they think is useful may actually irritate you. I had someone offer to drive with me to my VT sessions, but she wouldn't be quiet and made my driving experience all the more challenging. Others, upon hearing that merging traffic is hard for you, may become annoying backseat drivers when they are in your car, giving you too many driving directions when you don't need them. Your reaction might be to get annoyed or angry. You have to realize that they don't know what to do to help you. Even that annoying aunt who brings a big bag of carrots at family gatherings to "help your eyes" and gives you a disposable camera so you can take photos of what you see so she can understand what you mean by the "beauty of seeing some-one with two noses," is, in her way, trying to help, even if her actions may seem asinine and annoying.

Friends might invite you to inappropriate events and venues because they want to be inclusive and not make you feel left out, while you may be irritated by what you perceive as their insensitivity. While in some cases they may truly be careless and insensitive, if they are doing it to be inclusive and because they think that sometimes you may be able to go out dancing in a loud place at night or play miniature golf, then you may need to be clearer to them about what you can and cannot do.

Be open and direct about what you need. If you need your friends to help you parallel park your car when approaching their neighborhood with bad street parking, tell them that you'll call them when you're approaching their house so they'll be outside and ready to help you.

Your limitations are a completely foreign concept to most people you'll encounter in your life. It's your responsibility to be as clear as possible.

12. Your optometrist is not your psychologist.

Although your optometrist may be the only person you know who understands what VT is, they are not trained to be your counselor and may not have the time to help you deal with your non-visual side effects or past emotional trauma from surgeries, being mocked at as a kid, etc. Due to the scarcity of binocular vision specialists, these practitioners have busy offices.

13. Have a back-up plan.

Difficult sessions where you're pushing your eyes and brain to do what you have never done before can be so debilitating that driving home may make you a threat to society. Have a back-up plan. Figure out which public transportation you can take to get home or to a nearby friend's home to rest. Let your friends and family who live near your doctor's office know that you may call them last-minute if you need to rest at their house or spend the night in case you can't drive. Take a nap in your car and then get some food or drink before driving home.

14. Be open to learning new things about yourself.

When I decided to begin VT, I didn't know that as I awakened my brain to use both eyes, I was also going to learn things about myself that I previously didn't know.

Once I found out that not seeing in 3D made it hard for me to drive, I understood why my two strabismic aunts limited their driving to daytime hours and surface streets, avoiding the highway. Since driving is a common difficulty for people who don't see depth, some avoid driving altogether. Once I read more about depth perception, I understood why I drove so cautiously while others with "normal" vision didn't have to act in the same way.

Your small habitual ways of acting, which you may have never comprehended previously, will make sense.

When walking downstairs, I have always held the handrail to guide me while others would speedily run down the stairs hands-free. I have trouble seeing where one step ends and where another begins, especially in poor lighting. That's why I hold the handrail and look down while walking. I met a strabismic young lady in the lab who told me her mom would always rent ground floor apartments. When the woman was a child, she had trouble going up and down stairs.

If you ever felt inadequate while playing tennis, squash or some other sport requiring major hand-eye coordination, your limited depth perception may be a major factor in your troubles. When you can't see how far away something is when it is coming towards you, it's hard to position your racquet such that you hit the moving target. I've never heard of a Wimbledon champion who was born with asymmetric eyes.

These realizations are unlikely to come all at once. They may dawn on you while you wait for a bus one day or when someone makes a comment about your strange way of doing something that makes no sense to them. I still find myself uncovering new things about myself.

15. Ignorance is not bliss.

Most likely, when you tell people you can't see in 3D, they will tell you that they have never met anyone like you before. Unless you're talking to someone who has just been living the life of a recluse in a monastery and hasn't spoken to people for the past 20 years, you are not the first person from 2D land to have made their acquaintance. You're probably the first person to have opened your mouth and shared this information. Statistically speaking, one in every 33 people may have strabismus and/or amblyopia. Once I opened up about my visual condition, I found out that two of my close friends had also done VT for vision issues and had experienced diplopia and that my mom's distant cousin was also an amblyope.

It may take courage to speak up about your way of seeing the world to give others the space and comfort to confide in you and others about their limited depth perception.

We inspire others through our authenticity about who we are. You're not alone but if you keep quiet, you will feel terribly isolated. Keep in mind tip #1 about being careful with whom you share.

16. Give up the idea of being in control of your life.

I am not a Buddhist teacher or New Age spiritual leader. I am just speaking from the heart. The sooner you give up controlling your life, the easier it will be to accommodate the neural changes your brain is going through. The more you fight all the side effects (headaches, fatigue, double vision, confusion, over-sensitivity to sound, mood swings, etc.), the harder you make it for your brain to change.

If you're a control freak or even a closeted (hidden) one, deal with your control issues BEFORE you go to VT. I always considered myself a fairly flexible person as I've traveled and lived in many places where going with the flow was the only way to keep one's sanity, but life in VT has made me realize how much control and order I really like in my life.

Five years into VT, I still cancel events because of fatigue, headaches or other VT side effects.

This point cannot be overstated enough. When I finally surrendered myself to VT and said I'd find a way to manage the side effects and stop trying to lead my life the way I did before VT, it got easier.

It took me over three years in VT to realize that my own lack of acceptance of my reality and limitations was the cause of many of my problems. Previously, I had thought it was because other people didn't respect the therapy I was doing and my limitations and would still ask me to do things I couldn't do (like drive long distances at night). I still do get bothered by the actions of others, but I can't control their insensitivity or ignorance. The only thing I can control is my acceptance of myself and being able to surrender to the roller coaster of emotions and experiences along this path. If other people don't accept your limitations, that is their problem. Focus on what you can control: yourself. The sooner you are compassionate with yourself instead of seeking compassion or empathy from others, the sooner you will feel more comfortable with VT and your vision.

If you're not ready to modify your pace of life and how you socialize, then you are not ready for VT and to see anew.

Keep in mind, I've had two operations to surgically straighten my eyes. I am fighting against surgeries and scar tissue so my complications may be more severe than those who haven't been under the knife. But from what I've read online from other adults in VT, my symptoms are shared by others.

17. VT is like having your brain on crutches that nobody can see.

Vision therapy can be like physical therapy when you're re-learning to walk while on crutches, except it's for your brain and eyes. The crutches are not visible. Remember that. Some people may think you are a hypochondriac or that VT is an indulgence when you speak about the issues you have with limited depth perception and side effects from VT. Don't expect any empathy or sympathy, especially if your eyes look straight.

You may look normal and nobody can perceive you are undergoing major brain restructuring, but you are. Never forget that you're not the same person you were before you boarded the train to stereo-land.

I have to remind myself that although I want to do X activity, I need to be careful, bring someone with me in case something happens or leave early so I won't get tired. I've gone from being a free spirit to being super cautious.

18. Put some fun in your exercises.

Staring at quoit vectograms with red-green glasses can get old and boring real fast. I did some of my homework with *The Daily Show* or the *Colbert Report* in the background so I could listen to (not watch) comedians talk about current events while training my eyes. Tying your homework to listening to an audiobook, podcast or TV show may be a way to motivate you to do boring and repetitive homework. Play music that isn't too distracting.

19. Don't compare yourself to other patients.

If you see another patient move on to using prism glasses or the Brock string exercise before you do, that doesn't necessarily mean that you or your doctor are doing something wrong or that you are too slow. Patients vary widely from each other and each case is different. You may not know that the person who you think is progressing faster than you has another vision issue that may block him or her in a different way. If you worry about comparing yourself to others, you will only frustrate yourself even more.

20. Binocular vision problems don't define who you are.

Having amblyopia can make life difficult: VT can tire you, cost a lot of money and occupy much of your time. To make your life more enjoyable, find activities that you can enjoy alone or with friends that don't tax your visual system.

Despite being stereblind, I've written three books, supervised three book translations and have made a documentary film, even with tape on my glasses! If you have dreams, don't let your depth perception stop you.

21. If you need to do group activities, VT may not be for you.

All VT exercises are solitary marathons and competitions with yourself. The vision therapist or eye doctor will be near you but you have no team activities. Unless you have kids near you or very open minded and supportive adult friends and family with whom to do your homework, you will be on your lonesome every day while you work with the Brock String, tranaglyphs and other VT equipment. The only person with whom you can share your triumphs and pitfalls is your eye doctor or vision therapist. You have to become your own coach and cheerleader because your doctor will not be at your side all day, when you may be doing your homework, fighting off diplopia or trying to make sense of your changing vision. If you are not used to solo activities requiring self-discipline and motivation, read about how to motivate and pace yourself or speak to a psychologist about how to mentally set yourself up for this challenge.

22. Don't test new glasses on the road.

Don't drive home from the optical place with your new glasses. Wear them around at home first for a while, to get used to them in general. If you are trying prism glasses for the first time, they can be disorienting. You may try wearing them for just a few hours a day in a familiar place to get used to them. Only drive in new glasses once you are confident wearing them.

23. Make time for homework.

VT takes a lot of time outside of the actual sessions (30 minutes or an hour a day). You need to dedicate hours to the homework and make yourself be vigilant to do the work on your own.

24. Close your eyes in between exercises.

Your eyes and brain will tire easily in VT and with homework. Close your eyes for a few seconds or longer to let them rest, especially when you are concentrating on exercises with small targets. You may realize, upon taking a short break, that you will see better and feel a bit more refreshed after closing your eyes.

On parenting children with binocular vision issues

Parents of young children reading this, consider your children lucky. You are giving your kid(s) the chance to see straight and in 3D and not have to go through the difficulties of those of us doing VT as adults. When you are a child, it is easier for your brain to assimilate new behavior. Even though research has shown that the brain is more elastic than previously thought, it is hard to teach an old dog new tricks. Not that I was old when I commenced VT, but my brain had not been using the images from both of my eyes for over three decades. I had become a master suppresser, not even realizing when I was suppressing the vision from my left eye. One of the reasons I struggled so much in VT was that my brain didn't want to stop blocking what I was seeing in my left eye. A younger patient may still have trouble and side effects, but they will most likely experience less of that than I did.

Believe it or not, some parents have no idea that their children lack depth perception. If their kids have only a small asymmetry in their eyes or don't have asymmetry at all and don't complain about their eyesight, parents may not realize that their kids can't see in 3D. Many think that if their children can read normally, then they are fine. Parents without health insurance may not be able to afford to take their child to an optometrist and/or ophthalmologist. In this case, the Lions Club gives free eye exams and eye glasses worldwide. When my parents were unemployed and couldn't afford to buy me glasses, they asked my elementary school for help. Via the local Lions Club, my school sent us to a local optometrist who did an exam, gave me a prescription for glasses and gave me a new pair of glasses. However, I was never told I couldn't see in 3D. Keep in mind that not all vision tests screen for binocularity issues.

If you are not sure if your child has amblyopia and/or strabismus, look out for these things:

1. If your child often tilts their head to the side, they may be doing this unconsciously, as I did and still do, in order to see better. Strabismics may tilt their heads to the position where their eyes see straighter.

2. If your child reads with one eye closed, they may be doing this to avoid seeing in double.

3. If your child complains that words "move" on the page when reading, their eyes are shifting around the page. This had happened to me throughout my life without my realizing that it had to do with strabismus. My eyes would jump from one line of text to another but it wasn't so bad that it prevented me from reading. For some strabismics, this constant "jumping" is so bad that they have trouble reading.

4. If your child writes in a slanted way on the page, without writing horizontally on the lines, and/or skips lines when writing, they may be doing this because their eyes are jumping around and they can't stay focused in one place.

5. If your child has limited verbal skills, you can offer invaluable observations of how your child accommodates visual limits in daily life. During the exam or therapy, you can help the doctor because you know how to best calm and encourage your child, and can help your child focus.

Vision therapy made me a stronger person

In the Russian language, there's a phrase for a question which is emotionally difficult to ask and answer: we call it a *больной вопрос* (bolnoy vopros), a "painful or sore question." There are three such "painful" questions I occasionally get from people brave enough to ask them.

1. **Would you have been better off not knowing that you could see only in 2D and that most of the world can see in 3D?**

   No. As painful of a realization as it was, finding out there was a reason why I was so poor at common activities like walking down stairs, parking a car, merging in traffic and other actions requiring depth-perception was a relief. I found out that it wasn't that I was dumb. I had a limitation which prevented me from performing these activities to the level expected for the majority of the population. Vision therapy has been a pathway for me to learn a great deal about myself and other people. In this case, ignorance is not bliss. I can't say I am living a blissful existence now, but awareness is power.

2. **Do you think you would still be so capable with foreign languages and hearing if it weren't for your visual disability?**

   Who knows? I do think that because of my impaired sight I pay much more attention to auditory cues, just like other people with disabilities who become very strong in their other senses.

3. Would you give up your languages for 3D vision?

This is a hypothetical question, so it is useless to pose it but nonetheless people do it anyway, probably to satisfy their own curiosity without taking into account that it's impossible for me to answer because I don't see in 3D yet. There's no answer. I am not giving up my language ability for something unknown.

All of these questions tie into my main insight about finding strength within myself, no matter whether people understood me or not. Being aware of my disability and accepting it, as in the last stage of grief, was a blessing.

The book, *David and Goliath: Underdogs, Misfits, and the Art of Battling Giants* by Malcolm Gladwell shows how advantageous disadvantages have helped people outperform their peers who don't have their disadvantage. The author shows how successful people who had to overcome hardships credit their disadvantages for their perseverance and success. Gladwell calls the disadvantages "desirable difficulties." He profiles a successful trial attorney who is dyslexic and made it through law school by memorizing case law. He grew up listening to his mother read him books at night and developed a precise oral memory. When he graduated from law school, he knew he couldn't be a judge's clerk or work in a law firm doing research because reading large amounts of information would be too hard. However, due to his strong capacity to listen to oral arguments, he honed his skills in the courtroom by listening carefully to people's testimony and catching them in their lies and mistakes. Gladwell correctly points out that not every dyslexic can jump over such hurdles as the successful people he highlights in his book. Some dyslexics don't get the attention they need in school to learn to read and therefore end up with few opportunities.

However, the premise of the book is fascinating, as are Gladwell's stories of people who, as the saying goes, "made lemonade out of lemons" and found a way to turn their disability or disadvantage into something that positively set them apart from the rest of their colleagues.

I have often wondered about how much my language skills and keen attention to auditory content are linked to my visual impairment. However, I have yet to meet other strabismic polyglots like myself. I can't be certain that my multilingualism is due only to my being strabismic but I do know that I pay much more attention to auditory input than most people around me, which has helped me learn music and languages.

Beyond my language capabilities, I truly believe that growing up with a noticeable eye turn before I was 17 gave me a level of inner strength that allows me to weather some difficult currents and storms. I discussed this with Vivian, another amblyopic lady in my town who is also doing vision therapy to develop 3D vision. Her grandmother used to call her retarded as a kid because of her wandering eye. She grew into being a tough girl at school that other kids avoided because she would get into fights. Although I wasn't a tough kid in school, Vivian and I share an inner resilience. Since we were mocked as children for our looks, we had to learn to tough it out on our own, seek our own paths and find medical professionals to help us improve our vision. We have both become super independent people who empathize with others who are ridiculed for looking different and who are isolated in some way. Sometimes people ask me where I get the psychological endurance to travel so much on my own, especially to difficult places. I started this independent path at a very young age, when I was two years old in the pre-school for the developmentally disabled. The 3% or more of us who can't see in 3D live in a world dominated by people who see in 3D with products and sports designed for those with "normal" vision. We have adapted to that world, consciously or unconsciously, and have had to find ways to live under the rules made by the majority. In my case, this ability to survive and sometimes thrive in conditions ill-suited for my limitations have made me seek out irregular and creative ways of life. I learned many languages, not only in the traditional way with books, but also with music, movies and television. I go for long walks, even in areas with uneven surfaces, but I do so with my head pointed to the ground so I can mind my step. Without fame or fortune on my side, I have found ways to get in the media to discuss my books and movie, by not being afraid of contacting many journalists directly and asking people to introduce me.

Vision therapy has strengthened my perseverance in pursuit of a goal and passion. Despite our sacrifices and hard work, unfortunately, we do not always get everything to which we aspire. Not striving for my development would be like giving up on life. I learned that I should always do my best, even if I don't completely reach my goal.

The past years of VT have fortified me in ways that I had never imagined. When you know that it is possible to see your walls vibrate, the lines on your floor move and your friend have two noses and three eyes, while you are completely sober, you tap into an awareness of the amazing power of the human brain to create what is not normally seen. I question what reality is because of the tricks my brain is playing when trying to protect me from seeing double.

The "small" improvements in my hand-eye coordination and vision mean that I am much better at my jump shot in basketball and I marvel at tree branches as I approach them. But these aren't the reasons someone would approach VT, especially given the costs involved with the therapy. Although I don't see in 3D yet, I do have better depth perception and acuity than before. I am still working on improving my depth perception in the lab at the UC Berkeley Optometry School. I haven't given up because

I am still noticing small improvements in my vision and I want to keep seeing progress.

What was most important to me was to learn about myself. Filtering through people in my life who mattered enough to me and who cared enough to truly listen and remember my limitations gave me insight into who I am and what is important to me. People with binocular vision issues don't go into VT with the intention of doing psychotherapy; they approach VT to improve their vision. Whether I develop more depth perception or not, I've gained something that I will not give up: knowing who I am at my core and appreciating what I have. My Spanish friend, Marilo, was right, VT made me into a different person.

Unfortunately, I am still living with the side effects of VT. Slowly, my energy levels returned to normal unless I was trying a new vision therapy exercise or the doctor made my exercises more difficult. In those cases, I could get tired and hungry, develop a headache and nausea all at once. The noise sensitivity did not get better, but the language confusion is not as bad as in my first year of VT. I still see the left lane on the highway double sometimes and I have to mentally block out the image of the extra left divider lane. My dancing in places with bright lights is still limited. I have accepted these as part of my life.

The goals I set out at the beginning of the book were to show what living with 2D vision is like and what VT is, to increase awareness of binocular vision issues, and to share the story of personal growth I experienced while improving my vision. I hope that if you are a fellow amblyope or have other binocular vision problems, that this book may have helped you feel less alone. Maybe this book will ease the road for others who pursue VT as they will know the pitfalls to avoid when communicating about their condition with those who see in 3D. If you are supporting a friend or family member with this condition, perhaps this book gave you more insight on how your friend/relative is dealing with the world and their changing brain and vision.

One of the readers of my blog contacted me to ask about vision therapy options near San Francisco and I told her about the lab at UC Berkeley. When I met her in the lab one day, she told me that her husband didn't understand how she could live without 3D vision and why she was dedicating so much time to the lab. I hoped that once my book was published, she could have her husband read it so he could understand her commitment to improving her vision. I was elated when I met her and left the lab grinning from ear to ear because I saw the impact that my blog had on her life. I realized I could help many more people be able to not only pursue their dreams to see better but also use this book to educate their family and friends about our condition.

I thought I was almost done with this book until I heard a song by Billy Joel as I was driving to UC Berkeley. Despite being a huge fan of Billy Joel's music, I don't listen to it often. The song, *The Stranger*, which I had heard many times before, but had never particularly taken interest in, spoke to me loud and clear, as though I were listening to it for the first time.

I replayed the song more than 10 times as I was walking around Berkeley, working to identify what exactly resonated with me on the theme of my vision. The sections below mirrored what I learned in the process of VT:

Well we all have a face *That we hide away forever*	When I was 17 and transformed into a "normal" looking teenager, I hid away my strabismic face. But I was always strabismic even though I had no idea that I couldn't see in 3D.

Though we share so many secrets
There are some we never tell
Why were you so surprised
That you never saw the stranger

Did you ever let your lover see
The stranger in yourself?
Don't be afraid to try again
Everyone goes south
Every now and then
You've done it, why can't someone else?
You should know by now
You've been there yourself

When I revealed my secret about my problematic vision, I exposed the stranger within myself to friends, lovers and family. It was only then that I could deem who cared enough to listen and remember who I really was and how I experienced the world. I know how hard it is to let others see the strabismic stranger inside oneself. But as the song says, "Don't be afraid to try again." Just pick the right people with whom to share your stranger.

Once I used to believe
I was such a great romancer
Then I came home to a woman
That I could not recognize
When I pressed her for a reason
She refused to even answer
It was then I felt the stranger
Kick me right between the eyes

I used to think I had many friends who truly cared about me. When I pursued my VT goals, I recognized some friends' bad character traits and habits. When I asked them to be kinder towards me, they couldn't do it. That stranger within me most definitely kicked me hard, so hard that it took me a long time to admit how blind I had been to my social reality.

You may never understand
How the stranger is inspired
But he isn't always evil
And he isn't always wrong
Though you drown in good
intentions
You will never quench the fire
You'll give in to your desire
When the stranger comes along.

Once I became aware of how much better my life was because my VT side effects had limited my social life, I realized that my strabismic side effects weren't so evil all the time. I would have never quenched my desire to know what 3D was unless I had gone through this therapy.

Find that stranger within yourself.

Resources

Options: surgery, prisms, vision therapy

There is no magic pill or easy solution for people with binocular vision issues. Each option has its plusses and minuses and must be considered before taking action. Even though surgery seems like the easiest choice, especially if one's goal is to have straight eyes and not to improve depth perception, there are serious side effects and possible negative outcomes to weigh.

Theories about beauty attest that symmetrical faces are perceived as more attractive in both males and females. People unconsciously see asymmetric faces as undesirable and not beautiful and therefore may shun those with strabismus. Caricatures and cartoons show stupid or evil people with asymmetric eyes.

Understanding motivations for surgery

For those of us with divergent eyes, we are aware when people look at us funny because of our eyes. Some kids get labeled as evil and retarded and feel that way about themselves into adulthood. I know an engineer in Silicon Valley with a Masters from the Massachusetts Institute of Technology (MIT) who had a lazy eye. As a manager in a top engineering role, he was uncomfortable supervising employees who saw his asymmetric eyes. He felt that his employees looked at him like he was an idiot. He wanted to be taken seriously. He undertook surgery as an adult with the goal of appearing normal. People who have jobs where they have to look at other people have a good reason for wanting to appear "normal." I would not have felt as comfortable doing TV interviews and presentations if my eyes didn't appear straight.

If you have a child who feels ridiculed or undesired because of their eyes, you must understand that even if you unconditionally love your child and accept them with their divergent eyes, the rest of the world may not. You must take seriously your child's desire to look "normal" and carefully consider the pros and cons of surgery, VT and prism glasses. The same goes for adults who are overcoming their fears of getting surgery or doing VT to straighten their eyes.

Does this mean that everyone with eyes that aren't straight should go on the operating table? Absolutely not. I know people whose eyes aren't straight and they don't want surgery. They are fine with the way they are.

The US ophthalmologists were in shock that I hadn't been operated on yet when I came to the US at the age of three. My parents agreed to my first surgery. They were operating with insufficient information because the option of binocular vision therapy was not even offered.

My parents had no clue about VT when I got my surgeries at ages three and 17. I was the one who asked for the surgery at 17 to straighten out my wandering eye.

I have no regret for having been under the knife because having straight-looking eyes for the last half of my life has been a blessing.

Those who have not had surgery to straighten their eyes have an easier time than I do with vision therapy because they have no scar tissue and shortened muscles. I am very aware that those two operations are making my VT progress difficult and slow. Some optometrists will not do VT on patients who have had surgery.

Those who didn't have surgery may have experienced severe humiliation and social isolation because of their wandering eye(s). I do know of people who have opted not to do surgery and found ways to overcome the stares or strange comments.

Commenter #7 says:

Hi there. I like your post and blog. I had surgery when I was 35 to correct an alternating divergent exotropia. I struggled for years with the decision to have it, but I can tell you five years later, with no "relapse," it's been worth it. The emotional wound is still there, and every time I read stories about the social isolation and constant rejection strabismus can cause, my chest constricts and I want to cry. For me, strabismus surgery was an imperfect solution for an imperfect world. Choose your challenge. Choose your struggle.

The decision whether to take the risk of surgery is a personal one.

For parents deciding whether to submit their children to surgery, I have no easy solution for your quandary. Please consider all of the options carefully.

Surgery

Surgery to cosmetically straighten the eyes of a strabismic person aims only to make the eyes appear straighter. The eyes will likely still be partially misaligned either vertically or horizontally. Operations do **not** give strabismic people 3D vision.

Pros: Unless there are complications, patients are in and out of the hospital within a day. Surgeries are done under general anesthesia.

Cons: As with any surgery, the risk of death is always present. Some patients say their eyes looked worse after surgery than before. Some people reported that they have terrible double vision after their surgeries. It can take more than one surgery for someone's eyes to appear straight. As one ages, the eyes may stray again, requiring another surgery if one wants to keep the eyes looking straight. If you want to do vision therapy after surgery, you may have the added challenge of working against the scar tissue from the surgery.

Find out more about strabismus surgery here: http://www.aapos. org/terms/conditions/102.

Only an ophthalmologist, a medical doctor (MD), can perform strabismus surgery. Often times, strabismus specialists are pediatric ophthalmologists.

Prism glasses

Pros: Prism glasses have horizontal and/or vertical prisms forcing the eyes to look "straight." Most strabismics in VT have to wear prism glasses, especially for their vertical misalignment, to force their eyes to be straight and for the brain to fuse the images from both eyes.

Cons: Some vision insurance plans don't cover prism lenses, only standard lenses, meaning you may have to pay $100 or more for the lenses out-of-pocket. Prism lenses can be heavy, leaving indentation marks on your nose. I suggest paying for the extra-thin lenses. Opticians not trained in strabismus could order you the wrong glasses. (It happened to me and I describe in it in the "Advice on Purchasing prism eye glasses" section.) Don't order prism glasses online because the prescription is delicate and requires special attention. You need to go to a lens shop where the people are trained in how to deal with difficult prescriptions.

I have met only one adult who got bad double vision from experimental prism glasses she got as a kid. I think her case is highly rare.

Vision therapy (VT)

Pros: You can straighten your eyes and improve your vision simultaneously. Some people might be able to straighten their eyes without surgery just by doing VT or by doing VT and wearing prism glasses. Others may need a combination of surgery, VT and maybe also prism lenses.

Cons: Double vision, fatigue, headaches, nausea, noise sensitivity and other side effects. Few insurance plans cover vision therapy in the US. If you're in a remote area, it can be difficult to find a trained doctor. Doing VT at home without doctor supervision could result in double vision or in other visual problems you don't know how to reverse on your own.

To find an optometrist trained in binocular vision therapy: http://www.covd.org

CAUTION, ACHTUNG, AVISO, ВНИМАНИЕ:

Do not pursue VT on your own by playing 3D video games and apps or watching 3D movies with an Oculus Rift, Zeiss VR One, Google Cardboard or another virtual reality device. It is tempting to save money and do vision therapy on your own by making your own Brock string and other exercises. Do-it-yourself VT may come with a price. Not every person with binocular vision problems can be helped with VT. You need to be evaluated by a professional. An optometrist specialized in 3D video games for amblyopia told me that video games on virtual reality devices for patients with amblyopia should be considered as medical devices, not entertainment. If you're not under the supervision of an eye doctor and you develop double vision from playing a 3D video game, you will most likely not know what to do to stop the double vision. If you try driving after playing a video game, you could be a danger to yourself and society because of the fatigue, headaches and nausea these games can induce. Even people with 3D vision can experience fatigue and nausea from 3D video games, movies and apps.

Books:

Fixing My Gaze: A Scientist's Journey Into Seeing in Three Dimensions by Professor Sue Barry

Barry reports on how she developed 3D vision in her 40s by doing vision therapy. The book was #4 on Amazon's list of science books in 2009. Dr. Barry's story inspired me to embark on this journey. She explains both the scientific background for her neurobiological changes as well as how her vision changed.

I am very grateful for Sue Barry's courage to share her journey to see in 3D. I have read the book twice. Dr. Barry chronicles an intensely personal story of her journey from 2D to 3D. As a neurobiologist, she illuminates the science of brain elasticity and its relation to binocularity.

Fixing My Gaze is also available as an audiobook.

Living Well with a Hidden Disability: Transcending Doubts and Shame and Reclaiming Your Life by Stacy Taylor and Robert Epstein

This book is not geared towards amblyopia or VT but it is for anyone with a hidden disability, offering strategies for managing pain and flare-ups and dealing with confusing emotions. The author is a therapist who has a hidden disability. With her counseling background, she understands the range of emotions people experience when dealing with health situations that baffle the patient, medical professionals and the people closest to the patient.

I so wish I had read this book before I had started vision therapy as it would have saved me a lot of heartache and anguish over how to deal with other people's reactions and my own sense of self-worth. I probably would not have found several friendships ruined or strained because of friends' lack of understanding or respect for my experience and side effects. If you're struggling with how to be and how to manage other people in your life (friends, romantic partners, spouse, colleagues, therapists, doctors, etc.) in relation to your eye issues, I highly recommend this book.

The Mind's Eye by Dr. Oliver Sacks

In the chapter *Persistence of Vision*, Dr. Sacks recounts how his vision changed from 3D to 2D as a result of a cancerous tumor. In another chapter, "Stereo Sue," he tells the story of Sue Barry's entry into 3D vision. He also has stories of face blindness and other visual disorders and how they affect the lives of those who have them.

Article:

A Neurologist's Notebook, *New Yorker* Magazine June 19, 2006

"Stereo Sue": Why two eyes are better than one. By Oliver Sacks

http://www.newyorker.com/magazine/2006/06/19/stereo-sue

This is the first article I had read about Sue Barry's amazing journey into 3D vision via VT. It changed my life indefinitely.

Radio interview:

Fresh Air, National Public Radio. August 16, 2010

Do You See What I See? A Scientist's Journey Into 3D

http://www.npr.org/templates/story/story.php?storyId=128977924

This is Professor Sue Barry's interview with Terry Gross about gaining 3D vision.

Video:

Susan R. Barry, Professor of Biological Sciences at Mount Holyoke College, South Hadley, Massachusetts talks about *Fixing My Gaze* in this TEDx talk at Pioneer Valley.

February 2012

https://www.youtube.com/watch?v=XCCtphdXhq8

Websites/Internet Support Groups for VT, amblyopia and strabismus:

Both of these online groups were highly valuable. I learned from and connected with others.

Sovoto

Sovoto is a public forum, created to bring together everyone who wants to expand awareness and understanding for the impact of developmental vision problems upon lives.

www.sovoto.com

Eyes Apart Yahoo Group

A place for adults, teens, and parents of children with strabismus (squint, crossed eyes, lazy eye and amblyopia), to discuss knowledge, experiences, problems, and ideas related to strabismus.

https://groups.yahoo.com/neo/groups/eyesapart/info

Free eye exam:

If you can't afford an eye exam, contact your local Lions Club for help. They may organize a free vision screening in your area. They don't offer VT as part of their free services but you could ask for an exam and a glasses prescription. Ask if they can screen you for binocular vision problems.

http://www.lionsclubs.org

If you are not located near a Lions Club, look for a local optometry school to see if they have any community clinics at a free or reduced cost.

Questions to ask a developmental optometrist about potential treatment:

1. What are the possible side effects?

2. Have you dealt with a patient with similar circumstances? (Keep in mind that no two patients are identical. Patients often have other ocular issues which affect their vision. However, it is good to know how much experience the doctor has, especially if you have a difficult case.)

3. If you have a difficult case, ask the doctor if there are certain thresholds you or your child have to cross in order for VT to be successful. Ask if it would make sense to consider not continuing with VT if you or your child don't cross that threshold after a certain period of time. When I first started VT, my doctor said that if I didn't break down some of my ARC within a certain number of visits, he would refund part of my money if I stopped VT.

4. What do I, as a parent, need to do with my child when I am in the office with him or her?

5. What kind of homework will I or my child have? Parents, ask if you need to help with the homework and what kind of encouragement your child needs.

6. If I start to see in double, what do I need to do to stop the diplopia if I am driving, reading or at work?

7. Will I or my child need to wear an eye patch? If so, could we limit it to home-use?

8. If you or your child has trouble reading because of double vision or words moving on the page, ask for specific exercises to help you track better while reading.

9. How long do you think I will be in VT and how many times a week do I need to come to the office?

10. If you live far away and want to buy VT equipment to use at home, ask the doctor to write a letter so you can order the equipment. Bernell Corporation will not sell VT equipment without a doctor's prescription.

Upon finishing this book, you may be inclined to send me your ocular history or that of your family member, asking if VT, surgery or prism glasses are the right choices for you or your relative. I am not a trained professional in vision care. Giving you medical advice would not only be illegal, but it would go against my personal integrity. You will have to make decisions about your medical options with the help of an optometrist trained in binocular vision therapy, an ophthalmologist specialized in binocular vision issues and perhaps also a neuro-ophthalmologist. If you'd like to consult with other people with binocular vision issues, please go to sovoto.com.

Glossary

acuity or visual acuity (VA)
Acuity refers to the clarity of vision and the finest detail/resolution that an individual is able to observe. Visual acuity is based on optical and neural factors: the sharpness of the retinal focus inside the eye, the health and functioning of the retina, and the sensitivity of the visual cortex of the brain.

alternating vision
In patients with strabismus, they will fixate with only one eye at a time while the other is deviated away from the direction of focus. The brain will process vision from the fixating eye while suppressing the other. With alternating vision, patients switch which eye is fixating.

An alternator is always suppressing one or the other. I am a quick alternator. Most of the time, I am unaware which eye I am using.

amblyopia
Amblyopia (pronounced: amblee-o-pee-ah) (also called lazy eye) is a disorder of sight. This is a developmental problem that results as a compensating mechanism to prevent diplopia. There is decreased vision in one eye that is usually independent of anatomical damage in the eye or visual pathways. This is correctable if caught early. This is usually uncorrectable by eyeglasses or contact lenses.

There are five types of amblyopia: deprivation amblyopia (from congenital cataracts present at birth), anisometropic, meridional, refractive and strabismic amblyopia.

It involves decreased vision in an eye that otherwise appears normal.

In amblyopia, visual stimulation either fails to be or is poorly transmitted through the optic nerve to the brain for a continuous period of time. It can also occur when the brain "turns off" the visual processing of one eye to prevent double-vision, for example in strabismus (crossed eyes). It often occurs during early childhood and results in poor or blurry vision.

amblyoscope (also called haploscope and stereoscope)
The amblyoscope is an optical device for presenting one image to one eye and another image to the other eye. Usually, amblyoscopes use front-surfaced mirrors placed at different angles close to the eyes to reflect the images into the eyes.

ARC
Abnormal retinal correspondence (ARC), also anomalous retinal correspondence, is binocular sensory adaptation to compensate for long-standing eye deviation. The fovea of the straight (non-deviated) eye and non-foveal retinal point of the deviated eye work together, sometimes permitting single binocular vision.

astigmatism
An astigmatism causes blurred or distorted vision. It is caused by the irregular shape of the cornea or the lens inside the eye.

Bernell Mirror Stereoscope (Bat Wing)
This is a Wheatstone-type stereoscope, also called a Bat Wing. It trains a patient to diverge and converge. It can also be re-arranged as a cheiroscope. The patient has to use both eyes to see the images reflected in the two mirrors in order to fuse the two images into one. The device gets patients who have difficulty making convergent or divergent eye movements stretch their limits.

Brock string
A Brock string is a heavy cord with colored beads that is an inexpensive home use instrument for training the eyes to see near and into the distance. It utilizes physical diplopia for training suppression, binocularity and spatial localization.

central fusion
When the eyes are straight and the brain fuses images seen in the center of the person's vision.

convergence
Where the eyes turn in towards the nose. We naturally do this while looking at close objects. Convergence is the coordinated movement and focus of our eyes inward. Close work requires us to focus both of our eyes inward on objects that are near, including books, papers, phone devices, etc.

convergence insufficiency or convergence disorder
This is a sensory and neuromuscular anomaly of the binocular vision system, characterized by a reduced ability of the eyes to turn towards each other, or sustain convergence.

When we are not able to converge our eyes easily and accurately, problems may develop, such as: eye strain, headaches, double vision, difficulty reading and concentrating, avoidance of near work, poor sports performance and dizziness or motion sickness.

diplopia (double vision)
Diplopia is the simultaneous perception of two images of a single object. One image is of the object in its correct location and the other image can be of the object rotated, in a diagonal position or moved horizontally or vertically.

dioptre (UK), or diopter (US)
This is a unit of measurement to describe the optical power of a lens. These measurements correspond to how much light is bent. The higher the power, the shorter the distance it takes to

bend light a predicted amount. This distance is determined by taking the reciprocal of the dioptric power, which also corresponds to the focal length of the lens.

There is a difference between "diopters" and "prism diopters."

divergence

Divergence is the simultaneous outward movement of both eyes away from each other, usually in an effort to maintain single binocular vision when viewing an object. It is a type of vergence eye movement.

esotropia

Esotropia, commonly called crossed eyes, is the visual condition in which a person uses only one eye to look at an object while the other eye turns inward. Esotropia is a type of strabismus. This condition usually does not involve faulty or damaged eye muscles. Eye coordination may not be developed enough to provide normal control of the person's binocular vision.

exotropia

Exotropia, commonly called wandering eye, wall-eye or a divergent squint, is the visual condition in which a person uses only one eye to look at an object while the other eye turns outward. It is a form of strabismus and the opposite of esotropia. People with exotropia often experience crossed diplopia. The deviated eye is turned in or "crossed" when using the two eyes together.

far-sightedness

Hyperopia or hypermetropia is known as being far-sighted (US) or longsighted (UK). This is caused by an imperfection in the eye (often when the eyeball is too short or the lens cannot become round enough), resulting in difficulty focusing on near objects, and in extreme cases, a sufferer might not be able to focus on objects at any distance.

Horror fusionis

This is a condition in which the eyes have an unsteady deviation. The extraocular muscles make spasm-like movements that continuously shift the eyes away from the one single position where they would both be pointing, generating double vision. The name *horror fusionis* (Latin "fear of fusion") connotes that the brain appears to be actively preventing binocular fusion.

motion parallax

Parallax is a displacement or difference in the apparent position of an object viewed along two different lines of sight, and is measured by the angle or semi-angle of inclination between those two lines.

We use these cues in combination with prior expectations to determine the position and depth of objects. Objects that are far away will not move as much as near objects when we move our perspective. We will observe more motion parallax or displacement of a near object versus a distant object when we move the same amount.

near-sightedness (myopia)

Myopia, known as near-sightedness (US) and short-sightedness (UK), is a condition of the eye where the light that comes in does not directly focus on the retina but in front of it, causing the image that one sees when looking at a distant object to be out of focus, but in focus when looking at a close object. This condition could result from the eye having too much power, thus focusing light in front of the retina.

ophthalmologist

An ophthalmologist is a medical doctor specializing in medical and surgical eye problems and eye diseases.

optician

An optician, or dispensing optician designs, fits and dispenses corrective lenses. Opticians determine the specifications of various ophthalmic appliances to give the necessary correction to a person's eyesight. Some registered or licensed opticians manufacture lenses to their own specifications and design and produce frames and other devices.

optometrist

Optometrists are concerned with the eyes, vision, visual systems, and vision information processing. Optometrists (known as ophthalmic opticians outside the United States and Canada) prescribe and fit lenses to improve vision. In some countries, they are trained to diagnose and treat eye diseases. A behavioral or developmental optometrist is specifically trained to do vision therapy for binocular vision disorders, convergence insufficiency and other optometric disorders.

peripheral fusion

When the brain can fuse the vision seen in the periphery of the visual field.

polarized lenses (Polaroid lenses)

Polaroid glasses are used with vectograms or vectographic slides when doing stereopsis testing or training. Polaroid lenses allow testing where one part of the image is seen by only the left lens and another is seen by only the right lens. When viewed binocularly, both images are seen as one. You can also create 3D illusions when viewed binocularly, or the illusion of depth.

prism

A prism is a transparent optical element usually made of glass, plastic and fluorite that has flat, polished surfaces that refract light. At least two of the flat surfaces must have an angle between them. Prisms can be made from any material that is transparent to the wavelengths for which they are designed.

prism training goggles

Allow the patient to train without instruments while reading, working, etc. Prisms goggles allow you to shift the field of vision in each eye. For example, a patient who has suffered a traumatic brain injury may result in a visual field shift. In patients experiencing a shift they may have issues with balance, as well as simple activities such as walking in a straight line. Prism goggles can be used as a diagnostic aid to try and correct the patient's field shift to bring it back to their natural midline. In some cases, patients who have been unable to stand or to walk down a hallway without leaning on a wall are able to perform these activities again with the assistance of a prism.

red-green glasses
The right eye sees through the red lens and the left eye sees through the green lens. The user knows that both eyes are being used when they can see the anaglyphic images through both eyes. If they suppress one eye, then they will not be able to see the complete image.

strabismus
Strabismus (pronounced: strah-biz-mus), or crossed eyes, is the inability to direct both eyes towards the same fixation point. One eye may appear to turn in (esotropia), out (exotropia), up (hypertropia), or down (hypotropia). The eye turn may occur constantly or only intermittently. Eye-turning may change from one eye to the other (alternating strabismus), and may appear only when a person is tired or has done a lot of reading (decompensated phoria). Strabismus may cause double vision. To avoid seeing double, vision in one eye may be ignored or suppressed resulting in a lazy eye (amblyopia).

Strabismus is a condition in which the eyes are not properly aligned with each other. It typically involves a lack of coordination between the extraocular muscles, which prevents bringing the gaze of each eye to the same point in space, which thus hampers proper binocular vision, and which may adversely affect depth perception.

Amblyopia is a condition caused by strabismus or other amblyogenic factors.

stereopsis

Stereopsis is the perception of depth and three-dimensional structure obtained on the basis of visual information deriving from two eyes by individuals with binocular vision. The eyes are located at different lateral positions on the head. Therefore, binocular vision results in two slightly different images projected to the retinas. The differences are mainly in the relative horizontal position of objects in the two images. These positional differences are referred to as binocular disparities and are processed in the visual cortex of the brain to yield depth perception.

suppression of vision

Suppression of the vision from an eye is a subconscious adaptation to eliminate double vision. The brain will process the vision from one eye and ignore the vision from the other one.

tranaglyph (Bernell)

Variable prismatic red-green slides help build initial fusional reserves through peripheral and central fusion as well as stereopsis. Effective home training slides feature red-green targets on transparent vinyl.

vectogram/vectograph

A vectogram is a polarized stereogram (stereo images) consisting of two polarized images at right angles to each other. When viewed through polarizing lenses it presents one image to one eye and another image to the other eye.

A vectograph is a polarizing filter sheet that encodes a photographic image as areas which polarize light more or less strongly, corresponding to the darker and lighter areas of the image. When the sheet is viewed by itself in ordinary light, a pale image is seen.

If two such images, made to polarize in opposite directions and each encoding one of the images of a stereoscopic pair, are superimposed and viewed through glasses containing appropriately oriented polarizing filters, each eye sees only one of the images and a single three-dimensional image is perceived by people with normal stereoscopic vision.

vision therapy
Vision therapy is like physical therapy for the eyes and the brain, providing medically necessary treatment for diagnosed visual dysfunctions, preventing the development of visual problems and/or or enhancing visual performance.

Glossary

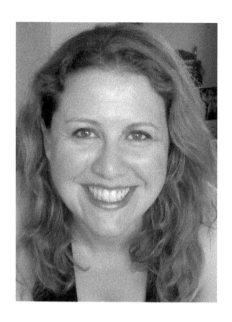

Susanna Zaraysky was born in Leningrad (in the former Soviet Union) with crossed eyes (strabismus) and came to the US as a young child. She received her first surgery for her asymmetric eyes in St. Louis, Missouri at the age of three and the second one in Santa Clara, California at the age of 17. Inspired by Professor Sue Barry's book, *Fixing My Gaze*, Susanna commenced binocular vision therapy in 2010 with the goal of seeing in depth.

She is a polyglot and author of the books *Language is Music* (translated in Portuguese, Russian and Spanish) on language learning via music and the media and *Travel Happy, Budget Low* on budget travel. Susanna is the co-producer of the documentary *Saved by Language*.

While going through vision therapy, Susanna hosted her own segment in Spanish on the *Al Despertar* morning show on Univision San Francisco called *El idioma es música* where she taught English grammar and pronunciation via songs. As an internationally known speaker on language learning, Susanna has given presentations in Bosnia, Cuba, Denmark, Kyrgyzstan, Laos, Mexico, Qatar and Russia, as well as at US universities, TEDx Santa Cruz and the US Defense and State Departments.

CBS, CNN, MTV, the BBC, The Guardian, the Filipino Channel, Yahoo Finance, Fox Business News, Univison, Telefutura, and MSNBC have interviewed Susanna on language learning and travel topics.

Works cited:

American Association for Pediatric Ophthalmology and Strabismus, article on strabismus, http://www.aapos.org/terms/conditions/100.

American Optometric Association, article on amblyopia, http://www.aoa.org/patients-and-public/eye-and-vision-problems/glossary-of-eye-and-vision-conditions/amblyopia/amblyopia-faqs?sso=y

Barry, Susan R. *Fixing My Gaze: A Scientist's Journey into Seeing in Three Dimensions.* New York: Basic Books, 2009.

Livingstone, Margaret. "The Power of the Image." In *Forum.* BBC. June 6, 2011. http://www.bbc.co.uk/programmes/poohcs2d

Kitaoji, H., and K. Toyama. "Preservation of Position and Motion Stereopsis in Strabismic Subjects." *Investigative Ophthalmology & Visual Science* Vol.28 (1987): 1260-267. Accessed September 26, 2015. doi:. http://iovs.arvojournals.org/article.aspx?articleid=2160004

Kübler-Ross, Elisabeth. *On Death and Dying.* 1969.

Sacks, Oliver. *Musicophilia: Tales of Music and the Brain.* New York: Alfred A. Knopf, 2007.

Sacks, Oliver. *The Mind's Eye.* New York: Alfred A. Knopf, 2010.

Sacks, Oliver. ""Stereo Sue": Why Two Eyes Are Better than One." *New Yorker Magazine,* June 19, 2006. http://www.newyorker.com/magazine/2006/06/19/stereo-sue

Taylor, Stacy, and Robert Epstein. *Living Well with a Hidden Disability: Transcending Doubt and Shame and Reclaiming Your Life.* Oakland, Calif.: New Harbinger, 1999.

Index

Symbols

A

B

C

M

Mind's Eye 19, 271
motion parallax 84, 280
myopia 280

N

near-sightedeness 280
New Yorker 7, 8, 13, 31, 39, 72, 271
Nobel Prize 48, 49, 126

O

ophthalmologist 7, 38, 57, 69, 112, 129, 146, 149, 176, 178, 207, 212, 217, 231,
    254, 265, 267, 275, 280
Oprah 159
optician 217, 219, 280, 281
optometrist 24, 30, 40, 50, 54, 57, 63, 84, 86, 91, 112, 115, 118, 119, 120, 125,
    128, 135, 149, 165, 167, 178, 195, 197, 202, 203, 207, 210, 213, 217, 218, 219,
    223, 231, 234, 242, 247, 254, 265, 268, 274, 275, 281

P

peripheral fusion 60, 281
Picasso, Pablo 143, 144
polarized lenses 61, 281
Princeton University 48
prism 61, 64, 65, 66, 88, 103, 114, 118, 120, 165, 217, 239, 245, 264, 267, 281
prism adapting/prism adaptation 120
prism training goggles 66, 108, 118, 120, 121, 165, 217, 218, 225, 230, 235, 245,
    251, 253, 265, 267, 275, 281

R

red-green glasses 45, 59, 61, 66, 69, 195, 231, 232, 251, 282
River of Dreams 53, 74, 142
Rodriguez, Silvio 155

S

Sacks, Oliver (MD) 7, 8, 31, 39, 72, 176, 182, 211, 271
Socrates 53
stereoblind 16, 18, 53, 72, 177, 202
stereopsis 102, 105, 202, 209, 242, 281, 283
stereoscope 277
Stereo Sue 7, 8, 13, 31, 39, 40, 45, 48, 72, 164, 211, 271

CPSIA information can be obtained
at www.ICGtesting.com
Printed in the USA
FSHW020731150919
62035FS